Physician's Guide to End-of-Life Care

For a catalogue of publications available from ACP–ASIM, contact:

Customer Service Center
American College of Physicians–American Society of Internal Medicine
190 N. Independence Mall West
Philadelphia, PA 19106-1572
215-351-2600
800-523-1546, ext. 2600

Visit our Web site at www.acponline.org

Physician's Guide to End-of-Life Care

Edited by

Lois Snyder, JD, and Timothy E. Quill, MD

for the American College of Physicians–American Society of Internal Medicine End-of-Life Care Consensus Panel

A|C|P

AMERICAN COLLEGE OF PHYSICIANS

PHILADELPHIA

Manager, Book Publishing: David Myers
Production Supervisor: Allan S. Kleinberg
Production Editor: Karen C. Nolan
Editorial Coordinator: Alicia Dillihay
Interior and Cover Design: Kate Nichols
Indexer: Dorothy Hoffman

Printed in the United States of America
Composition by Fulcrum Data Services, Inc.
Printing/binding by Versa Press

American College of Physicians (ACP) became an imprint of the American College of Physicians–American Society of Internal Medicine in July 1998.

PUBLISHER'S NOTE—Some of the chapters in this book originally appeared in *Annals of Internal Medicine* and *Journal of the American Medical Association.* They have been revised and expanded for book publication. See Journal Acknowledgements (page x) for complete bibliographical information.

Library of Congress Cataloging-in-Publication Data

American College of Physicians–American Society of Internal Medicine. End-of-Life Care Consensus Panel.
    Physician's guide to end-of-life care / edited by Lois Snyder and Timothy E. Quill for the American College of Physicians–American Society of Internal Medicine. End-of-Life Care Consensus Panel.
        p. ; cm.
    Includes bibliographical references and index.
    ISBN 1-930513-28-3
    1. Terminal care. 2. Physicians and patients. 3. Terminally ill--Care. 4. Hospice care.
I. Snyder, Lois, 1961- II. Quill, Timothy E. III. Title.
    [DNLM: 1. Terminal Care—methods. 2. Hospice Care—methods. 3. Palliative Care—methods. 4. Physician-Patient Relations. WB 310 A512p 2001]
R726.8.A46 2001
616'.029—dc21   2001022336

03 04 05 / 9 8 7 6 5 4 3 2

Editors

Lois Snyder, JD
Director, Center for Ethics and
    Professionalism
American College of Physicians-
    American Society of Internal Medicine;
Adjunct Assistant Professor of Bioethics
University of Pennsylvania Center for
    Bioethics
Philadelphia, PA

Timothy E. Quill, MD
Professor of Medicine, Psychiatry, and
    Medical Humanities
Program for Biopsychosocial Studies
University of Rochester School of
    Medicine
Rochester, NY

Contributors

Janet L. Abrahm, MD
Director, Palliative Care Programs
Adult Psychosocial Oncology Division
Dana-Farber Cancer Institute
Boston, MA

Donald M. Berwick, MD, MPP
President & CEO
Institute for Healthcare Improvement
Boston, MA

Susan D. Block, MD
Chief, Adult Psychosocial Oncology
Dana Farber Cancer Institute
Boston, MA

Ira R. Byock, MD
Director, Palliative Care Services
University of Montana
Missoula, MT

Arthur Caplan, PhD
Director, Center for Bioethics
University of Pennsylvania
Philadelphia, PA

David J. Casarett, MD, MA
Philadelphia Veterans Affairs Medical Center
Instructor, Division of Geriatrics
Institute on Aging
Center for Bioethics
University of Pennsylvania
Philadelphia, PA

LaVera M. Crawley, MD
Lecturer in Medicine
Center for Biomedical Ethics
Stanford University School of Medicine
Palo Alto, CA

Lynn Etheredge, BA
Consultant
Health Insurance Reform Project
George Washington University
Washington, DC

Kathy Faber-Langendoen, MD
Director, Syracuse Program in Bioethics
Department of Medicine
Health Science Center
State University of New York
Syracuse, NY

Sharon K. Inouye, MD, MPH
Associate Professor of Medicine
Department of Internal Medicine
Yale University School of Medicine
New Haven, CT

Andrea Kabcenell, RN
Director, Breakthrough Series
    Collaboratives
Institute for Healthcare Improvement
Cornell University
Ithaca, NY

Jason H. T. Karlawish, MD
Assistant Professor of Medicine
Department of Medicine
Division of Geriatrics
Alzheimer's Disease Center
Institute on Aging
Center for Bioethics
University of Pennsylvania
Philadelphia, PA

Barbara A. Koenig, MD
Associate Professor of Medicine
Pulmonary & Critical Care Department
Center for Biomedical Ethics
Stanford University
Palo Alto, CA

Jean S. Kutner, MD
Assistant Professor
Division of General Internal Medicine
University of Colorado Health Sciences
    Center
Boulder, CO

Paul N. Lanken, MD
Professor of Medicine
Pulmonary & Critical Care Division
Department of Medicine
Center for Bioethics
University of Pennsylvania
Philadelphia, PA

Bernard Lo, MD
Professor of Medicine
University of California
San Francisco, CA

Joanne Lynn, MD, MA, MS
Director, Center to Improve Care of the
    Dying
George Washington University
RAND
Washington, DC

Patricia A. Marshall, MD
Associate Professor
Center for Biomedical Ethics
Case Western Reserve University School
    of Medicine
Cleveland, OH

Diane E. Meier, MD
Associate Professor
Departments of Geriatrics & Medicine
Mt. Sinai School of Medicine
New York, NY

Alan Meisel, JD
Director, Center for Bioethics & Health
    Law
University of Pittsburgh School of Law
Pittsburgh, PA

Kathleen Casey Milne, RN, CCM, CMC
Program Director
Center to Improve Care of the Dying
George Washington University
RAND
Washington, DC

Kevin Nolan, MA
Statistician
Associates in Process Improvement
Silver Spring, MD

Timothy E. Quill, MD
Professor of Medicine, Psychiatry, and
    Medical Humanities
Program for Biopsychosocial Studies
University of Rochester School of
    Medicine
Rochester, NY

Lois Snyder, JD
Director, Center for Ethics and
    Professionalism
American College of Physicians-
    American Society of Internal Medicine;
Adjunct Assistant Professor of Bioethics
University of Pennsylvania Center for
    Bioethics
Philadelphia, PA

James Tulsky, MD
Associate Professor of Medicine
Duke University;
Director, Program on the Medical
    Encounter & Palliative Care
VA Medical Center
Durham, NC

David Weissman, MD
Director of Palliative Medicine
Professor of Medicine
Medical College of Wisconsin
Milwaukee, WI

Anne Wilkinson, PhD
Senior Health Policy Analyst
The Center to Improve Care of the
  Dying
RAND
Washington, DC

Acknowledgements

Grant Support: The editors and the American College of Physicians-American Society of Internal Medicine End-of-Life Care Consensus Panel wish to thank the Greenwall Foundation for support of the development of the papers in the end-of-life care series. We would also like to thank the College for Commission on Professional and Hospital Activities funding in support of this book.

Members of the End-of-Life Care Consensus Panel: Bernard Lo, MD, FACP, Chair; Janet L. Abrahm, MD, FACP; Susan D. Block, MD; William Breitbart, MD; Ira R. Byock, MD; Kathy Faber-Langendoen, MD; Lloyd W. Kitchens, Jr., MD, FACP; Paul N. Lanken, MD, FACP; Joanne Lynn, MD, FACP; Diane E. Meier, MD, FACP; Timothy E. Quill, MD, FACP; George Thibault, MD, FACP; and James Tulsky, MD. Primary staff to the Panel were Lois Snyder, JD (Project Director), Jason T. Karlawish, MD, and David J. Casarett, MD.

Consensus panel papers were reviewed and approved by the College's Ethics and Human Rights Committee, although they do not represent official College policy. Members of the Ethics and Human Rights Committee were Risa Lavizzo-Mourey, MD, FACP, Chair; Lee J. Dunn, Jr., JD, LLM; David A. Fleming, MD, FACP; William E. Golden, MD, FACP; Susan Dorr Goold, MD; Vincent Herrin, MD; Jay A. Jacobson, MD, FACP; Joanne Lynn, MD, FACP; David W. Potts, MD, FACP; and Daniel P. Sulmasy, OFM, MD, PhD.

JOURNAL ACKNOWLEDGEMENTS

Earlier, shorter versions of the End-of-Life Care Consensus Panel publications appeared as:

Lo B, Quill TE, Tulsky J. Discussing palliative care with patients. Ann Intern Med. 1999;130:744-9. (Chapter 1)

Karlawish JHT, Quill TE, Meier DE. A consensus-based approach to providing palliative care to patients who lack decision-making capacity. Ann Intern Med. 1999;130:835-40. (Chapter 2)

Abrahm JL. Management of pain and spinal cord compression in patients with advanced cancer. Ann Intern Med. 1999;131:37-46. (Chapter 5)

Block SD. Assessing and managing depression in the terminally ill patient. Ann Intern Med. 2000;132:209-18. (Chapter 6)

Faber-Langendoen K, Lanken PN. Dying patients in the ICU: forgoing treatment, maintaining care. Ann Intern Med 2000;133:886-93. (Chapter 8)

Quill TE, Byock IR. Responding to intractable terminal suffering: the role of terminal sedation and voluntary refusal of food and fluids. Ann Intern Med. 2000;132:408-14. (Chapter 9)

Meisel A, Snyder L, Quill TE. Seven legal barriers to end-of-life care: myths, realities and grains of truth. JAMA. 2000;284:2495-501. (Chapter 11)

Contents

Introduction

TIMOTHY E. QUILL, MD • LOIS SNYDER, JD

Medicine demonstrates its passion and its potential in the vigorous, technological fight against disease, and it has been remarkably successful. Because of this, and public health measures, people in the developed world are living longer. Many diseases that were uniformly fatal 20 years ago are almost routinely cured with modern treatments. Previously lethal infections are now regularly treated in primary care offices, almost without a second thought. The average life span for women is in the mid-80's, and in the upper 70's for men. What could possibly be wrong with this picture?

Unfortunately, there is a downside to these successes. Instead of dying quickly of acute illnesses such as infections, people die at the end of long chronic illnesses, often with physical and emotional suffering, debility, and dependence. Individuals and families struggle with whether, when, and how to stop treatment. The pneumonia that used to be "the old man's friend" is often reflexively treated with antibiotics, and the natural withdrawal from eating and drinking that occurs toward the end of life is countered with nutritional monitoring and feeding tubes. Modern medicine has demonstrated much less clarity and passion about how to address and relieve suffering toward the end of life, and patients, families, and doctors frequently struggle for answers about the daunting clinical and moral questions that arise in no small measure as a result of our ability to prolong life.

The evidence of inadequate access to and delivery of pain treatment and other palliative measures for seriously ill patients in the United States is clear and convincing (1,2). Pain and depression are under-recognized and under-treated in dying patients, and most physicians have never been trained to provide palliative measures. Medical training programs are only now beginning to address formal educational requirements in end-of-life care.

More than 40 million U.S. citizens are uninsured, lacking access to basic preventive care or ongoing care. They are at best treated episodically for emergencies that become too overwhelming to deny. Even with access to care, however, the SUPPORT Study demonstrated that access does not ensure adequate management of pain and other symptoms, nor does it ensure meaningful decision-making (3). This observational study of five teaching hospitals identified the common occurrence of prolonged deaths in intensive care units with poor understanding of patient preferences, inadequate pain management, and little effective end-of-life decision-making. A contemporaneous survey showed that physicians understood and were disturbed that they were over-using technology and under-treating pain but were uncertain about how to change (4).

The United States has an extensive system of hospice programs to serve terminally ill patients, provided they have acceptable insurance coverage, are expected to live 6 months or less, and are willing to forgo aggressive care (5). In the United States, hospice programs are largely home based, and usually require considerable involvement by family members to provide primary care, so hospice programs are not feasible for everyone. In many areas, there are a small number of residential hospice units, but they are inadequate to meet the needs of most communities. Unfortunately, patients with chronic diseases with uncertain prognoses (Alzheimer's disease, congestive heart failure, amyotrophic lateral sclerosis) who might otherwise benefit from hospice do not qualify (6). Only 25% to 35% of patients with cancer die in hospice programs, and referrals are often made very late in the course of the patient's illness, so often the opportunity to take full advantage of the program is lost (7,8).

Communication about end-of-life issues is itself very challenging, even for experienced clinicians (9). Physicians are reluctant to tell patients that they are likely to be approaching the end of their lives (10), and when they do discuss prognosis, they tend to be overly optimistic (11). This gap in relaying prognostic information accurately stems in part from medicine's inherent prognostic uncertainty (12), and from clinicians' feeling that they may be perceived as "giving up" on the patient if they talk about dying. Patients and families often collude in this avoidance and therefore passively accede to a continuation of potentially unwanted and ineffective technologic intervention, and lose an opportunity to address uncomfortable symptoms and to discuss matters of life closure.

Despite these inadequacies, there is a growing consensus about what good end-of-life care might look like, and there are many centers of excellence where it is beginning to be delivered (6). First and foremost, there is general agreement that acute, aggressive treatment of underlying disease need not preclude good palliative care, and that excellent treatment of pain, other physical symptoms, and other dimensions of suffering should be part of the treatment plan for all seriously ill patients, not just those who qualify for hospice or those who accept that they are actively dying. Thus, excellent pain and symptom management must be part of the armamentarium for all physicians who care for seriously ill patients, and patients should be able to count on state-of-the-art palliative treatment even when they are simultaneously involved in a vigorous, technology-dominated fight for life.

Furthermore, preparing psychologically, spiritually, and practically for the possibility of death does not preclude continuing with aggressive disease-directed treatment. Most clinicians would not think twice about recommending an invasive medical treatment with a 25% chance of cure, yet that same patient may have a 75% chance of dying sometime in the process of treatment. It might behoove such patients to hope and plan for the best, but to also take the opportunity to prepare for the worst in case things do not go well (which in this example is the most probable scenario.)

In the past, palliative care has been equated with hospice and has therefore been held in reserve for those who are relatively certain to die within 6 months, who accept this, and who are willing to forgo aggressive treatments. A more common clinical circumstance is patients who want to continue some or all aggressive treatments in the hope of prolonging survival, but might also benefit from palliative care measures. After all, these patients are still relatively likely to die in the near future, and, even if they don't, why not provide them with the best pain and symptom management? By asking the question, "Would you be surprised if the patient died in the next 6 months?" clinicians can identify a very different population than they would by asking, "Are you sure the patient will die within the next 6 months?"

Hospice care works with a relatively small subset of dying patients in which clinicians are relatively sure death will come in 6 months, and in which patients are willing to forgo aggressive treatments. Such patients must achieve some level of acceptance that they are dying before they are referred and must have relatively clear prognoses. More patients, however, do not meet the prognostic criteria, do not accept that they are likely to die in 6 months, or are unwilling to forgo aggressive treatment. Although such patients won't qualify for formal hospice programs, they will clearly benefit from palliative measures (pain and symptom management), they may want to make sure their affairs are in order (will and living will), and they may want to consider some of the developmental issues of life closure.

Palliative medicine may eventually become a specialty within medicine to further teaching and research, but it must also be a core clinical skill for all physicians who care for seriously ill patients. The chapters of this book were developed by members of the ACP-ASIM End-of-Life Care Consensus Panel, a group of experts in end-of-life care convened in 1997 by the College with the support of the Greenwall Foundation. Additional experts outside of the group contributed as authors when needed. We have been privileged to work with all of these dedicated individuals, and to represent the group effort as editors of this volume.

The charge of the Consensus Panel was to identify clinical, ethical, and public policy challenges in end-of-life care where improvement was desirable, to analyze and critically evaluate available evidence and guidelines, and to offer consensus recommendations on how to better address these problems. Our audience is clinicians, both generalists and subspecialists, who care for seriously ill patients. Most papers are illustrated by at least one clinical case study, and every effort is made to be simultaneously evidence-based (where there is empirical evidence), consensus-driven (by the panel of experts), and very practical (so that clinicians would find the papers clinically relevant).

Section I addresses communication and building relationships. It begins with a chapter exploring how and when to initiate the discussion about palliative care and provides practical ideas about what questions to ask and how to follow up on the initial inquiries. Ideas about how to initiate inquiry into the patient's values and spirituality are also introduced. The second chapter presents a strategy for building a consensus among clinicians, patient, and family when the patient loses the ability to speak for himself or herself. Unfortunately, patients have often lost this capacity after a long illness when end-of-life decision-making is at its most challenging. Chapter 3 explores the influence that culture may have on end-of-life discussions and presents ideas about how to bridge gaps that might exist within these dimensions, which might otherwise pose barriers to decision-making and relationship-building. We know that the meaning of these end-of-life discussions and of suffering may vary considerably between and within cultures, so clinicians need to make this exploration part of their process. The final chapter in this section explores the roles and responsibilities that a clinician has in the care of a dying patient and how he or she might become part of the hospice team and part of the patient's and family's world.

Section II presents practical, evidence-based approaches to common end-of-life problems. In each of these chapters, a real clinical case is followed over time to illustrate how the challenges in the subject area change as patients approach death. Chapter 5 follows a patient with advanced prostate cancer and demonstrates how to use opioids in different doses and by different routes and also how to take advantage of the advanced technology of pain management in some special pain situations. In Chapter 6, the recognition and treatment of depression in severely ill patients is explored, including the distinction between clinical depression and sadness, as well as how to evaluate patients for reversible depression who may express a wish to die. Pharmacologic therapies, including amphetamines, that are relevant to treating depression in the terminally ill are reviewed. Delirium, which can be very common as death approaches, is addressed in Chapter 7, which describes its recognition, how to tailor its workup to the clinical situation, and practical management strategies. Chapter 8 discusses decision-making about forgoing life-prolonging therapy in the intensive care unit and then gives guidance about how to anticipate and manage potentially challenging symptoms that might emerge (such as shortness of breath when withdrawing a ventilator.) Chapter 9 explores the role of two "last resort" interventions, voluntarily stopping eating and drinking and terminal sedation, in the context of terminal illness and severe, intractable suffering. The importance of treating severe symptoms at the end of life with knowledge, creativity, and commitment is illustrated. Chapter 10 closes this section, with a practical approach to addressing the grief and bereavement of family members. What is normal grief, and when does it become medically worrisome? What is the physician's proper role with the family after the patient has died?

Section III deals with legal, financial, and quality issues in end-of-life care. In Chapter 11, legal barriers, myths, and realities are presented in terms of advance directives, surrogate decision-making, high-dose pain medicine, stopping life supports, and physician-assisted suicide. Practical guidance is given about the current state of the law, which, despite physicians' fears, is generally not a major impediment to most types of end-of-life-care. The financing issues that are a major impediment to good end-of-life care are illustrated in Chapter 12. For those who qualify for and choose hospice care, there is a good range of services and supports, but for the many other dying patients whose needs are comparable but who don't qualify, the system is not working. In this chapter, innovative, practical policy strategies that might promote and finance high-quality end-of-life care to a broader range of patients are explored. Finally, Chapter 13 shows how quality improvement processes might be used to improve end-of-life care when a problem is identified at a particular institution or community. The cycle of identifying a problem, collecting data, experimenting with system-based change, and then re-collecting data is illustrated through a case scenario.

On behalf of the members of the ACP-ASIM End-of-Life Care Consensus Panel, we hope that the readers (trainees as well as experienced clinicians) find this book valuable. It may be especially useful to read particular chapters when a palliative care problem in the domain covered is encountered. The articles were designed to be of practical value and are clearly focused on the topic identified in the title. The references should provide more detailed access to primary data when this is desirable.

By working intensively with severely ill and dying patients and their families, clinicians can improve their skills at identifying and addressing palliative care problems in real time. As all clinicians improve their basic skills in palliative care, quality of care and quality of life for such patients will improve, whether they choose to continue an aggressive fight against their disease all the way through to their death, or whether at some point they decide to make palliation their primary objective and then enter a hospice program. In addition to improving our individual skills, we must also commit to improving the training in these dimensions for the next generation of physicians. Again, many of these chapters provide an excellent, practical overview for teaching some of the most important elements of palliative care. Finally, and equally importantly, we must all work together to develop systems of care that are capable of supporting excellence in palliative care for all seriously ill patients, not just those who meet the rather narrow criteria for admission to a hospice program.

We are indebted to the authors of this volume and to the members of the ACP-ASIM End-of-Life Care Consensus Panel and Ethics and Human Rights Committee for their hard work, dedication, good nature, and contributions to thoughtful debate. We would also like to thank the Greenwall Foundation for support of the development of the consensus panel papers, and the American College of Physicians–American Society for Internal Medicine, for Commission on Professional and Hospital Activities funding in support of this book.

Death will come to us all, so how can we improve the end of life and the process of dying? We must work together to recognize the challenges of end-of-life care, and to develop the highest quality systems of care that support those who are dying by enhancing the quality and meaning of life and helping patients to make fully informed decisions based on the best possible information. It is a complex task, but we can clearly accomplish it if we find the same passion for end-of-life care that we have found for other dimensions of medicine.

REFERENCES

1. Approaching Death: Improving Care at the End of Life. Washington, DC: National Academy Press; 1997.
2. **Quill TE, Meier DE, Block SD, Billings JA.** The debate over physician-assisted suicide: empirical data and convergent views. Ann Intern Med. 1998;128: 552-8.
3. **The SUPPORT Principal Investigators.** A controlled trial to improve care for seriously ill hospitalized patients. The study to understand pronoses and preferences for outcomes and risks of treatment (SUPPORT). JAMA. 1995;274: 1591-8.

4. **Solomon MZ, O'Donnell L, Jennings B, et al.** Decisions near the end of life: professional views on life-sustaining treatments. Am J Public Health. 1993;83: 14-23.
5. **Rhymes J.** Hospice care in America. JAMA. 1990;264:369-72.
6. **Christakis NA.** Timing of referral of terminally ill patients to an outpatient hospice. J Gen Intern Med. 1994;9:314-20.
7. **Christakis NA, Escarce JJ.** Survival of Medicare patients after enrollment in hospice programs. N Engl J Med. 1996;335:172-8.
8. **Quill TE.** Initiating end of life discussions with severely ill patients: addressing the elephant in the room. JAMA. 2000;284:2502-7.
9. **Christakis NA, Iwashyna TJ.** Attitude and self-reported practice regarding prognostication in a national sample of internists. Arch Intern Med. 1998;158: 2389-95.
10. **Christakis NA, Lamont E.** Extent and determinants of error in doctors' prognoses in terminally ill patients. BMJ. 2000;320:469-73.
11. **Lynn J, Harrell F Jr, Cohn F, et al.** Prognoses of seriously ill hospitalized patients on the days before death: implications for patient care and public policy. New Horizons. 1997;5:56-61.
12. **Lynn J.** Caring at the end of our lives. N Engl J Med. 1996; 335:201-2.

SECTION I

The Interview and Relationship Building

CHAPTER 1

Discussing Palliative Care with Patients

BERNARD LO, MD • TIMOTHY E. QUILL, MD •
JAMES TULSKY, MD

Many patients experience distressing symptoms at the end of life that can be relieved through palliative care. Palliative care, which focuses on comfort and psychosocial support, is a foundation for all health care. Early in disease, many patients choose to undergo surgery, chemotherapy, or other disease-oriented treatments; patients may trade short-term discomfort for the prospect of longer survival or a better quality of life.

As disease progresses, however, many patients choose not to make such tradeoffs and choose palliation as the paramount goal of care. In this context, palliative care encompasses not only relief of suffering but also helping patients come to terms with their mortality, to live their last days with as much grace and equanimity as possible. But, although palliation is an essential element of patient care, it has been discouraged by the reimbursement system and is at odds with our culture's tendency to deny death (1), in addition to the fact that physicians lack training and often struggle when discussing palliative care with patients and families.

This chapter suggests how to improve discussions about palliative care. Because there are few rigorous empirical studies of communication regarding palliative care, these suggestions are based on clinical experience and intuition, as well as analogy to research on doctor-

3

patient communication in other contexts (2). The chapter is structured around several common clinical questions. How can physicians raise the topic of palliative care? When should we discuss palliative care with patients? How can physicians respond to difficult patient statements and questions? How can we discuss palliative care while disease-remitting treatments are continued? Two hypothetical case scenarios illustrate how to discuss palliative care at all stages of serious, progressive chronic illness; use effective interview techniques; and respond to patient and family emotions.

How Can Physicians Raise the Topic of Palliative Care?

Case 1-1 illustrates an approach to introducing the topic of palliative care. Because patients may be reluctant to raise difficult, painful topics, physicians usually need to take the lead.

CASE 1-1. PATIENT WHOSE CANCER HAS SPREAD DESPITE CHEMOTHERAPY

A 54-year-old businessman had carcinoma of the colon with liver metastases that enlarged despite two regimens of chemotherapy. He was hospitalized because of bruises, oozing from venopuncture sites, and nosebleeds caused by disseminated intravascular coagulation secondary to cancer. His disseminated intravascular coagulation responded only partially to heparin. The patient's right upper quadrant abdominal pain was well controlled with opioids. During the hospitalization, he tripped while going to the bathroom, causing a laceration and ecchymoses around his eyes. The oncologist discussed experimental chemotherapy and the statistical prognosis for refractory metastatic colon cancer.

Because of the patient's poor prognosis, the physician also wanted to raise the issue of palliative care. How might this be done? As physicians, we could simply ask, "Tell me what is most important to you now." For this patient, spending time at home with his family was paramount. The physician might then ask, "How is your family managing?" The patient's 5-year-old daughter, for example, was frightened because of his bruises and black eyes. We could continue to ask open-ended questions to elicit the patient's needs and goals: "How do you feel when you see your daughter frightened?" "What would you like to say to her when she is frightened?" Alternatively, if the patient becomes tearful, we might say, "Does it make you sad to see her frightened? It's so important for you to be with her." This empathethic comment names the patient's underlying emotion and identifies its cause (3). Through such open-ended questions and empathetic comments, we can encourage further discussion and help the patient re-evaluate his goals and wishes for care.

> *The patient questioned the usefulness of further chemotherapy: "It's a long shot, isn't it?" The doctor replied, "Yes, it is, and chemotherapy has side effects as well." After a silence, he added, "I wish we had more effective chemotherapy, but there are many things we can do to make sure you're not suffering." The physician then asked the patient's wife about her concerns. She felt unable to handle major bleeding by herself at home and said she would call 911 if problems arose. Eliciting the wife's perspective allowed the physician to discuss how hospice care provides home visits on short notice for such events as major bleeding (4). It is prudent to involve family members in discussions regarding palliative care. Patients generally want close family involved in these discussions. As in this case, they may raise additional issues that need to be considered, and their cooperation is needed for some options for care.*

Elicit the Patient's Concerns About Illness, Goals, and Values

Starting with open-ended questions encourages patients to talk about what is most important to them. Understanding the patient's perspective is usually helpful before delivering information, providing support, or recommending a plan of care. Such understanding allows the physician to orient the discussion to the patient's concerns and values. Useful questions include:

- "What concerns you most about your illness?"
- "How is treatment going for you and your family?"
- "As you think about your illness, what is the best and the worst that might happen?"

- "What has been most difficult about this illness for you?"
- "What are your expectations about the future?"
- "What are your hopes for the future?"
- "As you think about the future, what is most important to you?"
- "Knowing what you do about your condition, what matters most to you now?"

Such open-ended questions are more useful in eliciting patient concerns, needs, and emotions than questions that can be answered "yes" or "no" (5). Building follow-up questions on the exact language used by the patient enables the physician to individualize subsequent discussions.

Many doctors focus discussions on clinical decisions that need to be made, and talk about palliative care only after a decision to limit life-prolonging interventions has been made (6). However, starting with open-ended questions about the patient's concerns, hopes, and goals may be more effective. Specific clinical decisions are often easier to make after the patient's concerns and goals are known. Furthermore, open-ended discussion can build trust and a richer relationship with the patient.

In such discussions, many physicians are reluctant to use terms like "hospice" because they imply that death is imminent (7). However, other terms, such as "supportive care," "comfort care," or "comprehensive care," may be misleading or ambiguous. In many cases, it will be possible simply to provide many elements of palliative care, starting with the questions suggested above, without labeling it.

Ask Directly About the Patient's Symptoms

A good opening question is "How is your illness limiting your activities?" After open-ended questions, physicians can ask for a "review of symptoms" of common problems. Specifically, doctors can ask about pain on a numeric scale, for example, 0 to 10 (8). Physicians also should ask about fatigue, shortness of breath, and symptoms specific to the site of the patient's illness. Screening for depression is essential because depression is common and often overlooked. The simple question "Are you depressed?" is an effective screening tool (9).

Some patients may deny physical symptoms or psychosocial distress. In such circumstances, we can gather information about the patient's needs indirectly by asking such questions as, "How is your family dealing with your illness?" "Have any family members or friends had a similar experience?"

Offer to Talk About the Spiritual Aspects of Dying

Most experts in palliative care believe that attention to spiritual and religious issues is an essential component of palliative care (10). However, the physician's role may be controversial. Some physicians believe that it is more important to attend to palliation of physical symptoms. Others point out that physicians, unlike clergy, have no special expertise in spiritual matters. In their view, the patient's own religious advisor or a chaplain is better suited than a doctor to suggest answers to spiritual questions and to provide the solace of religious rituals. We believe that it is important to offer patients the opportunity to come to terms with their mortality and to find some meaning in the final stage of their life. Physicians can screen for unaddressed spiritual concerns and help patients find ways to explore spiritual issues, if they so desire. Open-ended questions are useful to begin discussions:

- "What do you still want to accomplish during your life?"
- "What thoughts have you had about why you got this illness at this time?"
- "Is faith or spirituality important to you in this illness?" If the patient answers affirmatively, one might ask: "Who can help you deal with these faith concerns?" "Have you talked with this person?" "How could this conversation with that person start?"

As physicians, our goal can be to help patients clarify their own feelings and beliefs if they wish to do so. By listening attentively, the physician can relieve the patient's sense of isolation and show respect for the patient's explorations of difficult issues. Many patients near the end of life want to talk to their physicians about spiritual and existential issues. In a recent poll, 30% of respondents reported that if they were dying a doctor would be "comforting to them in many ways outside of medical attention" compared with 36% who reported that a member of the clergy would be comforting (11). For these patients, more direct questions may be useful:

- "What is your understanding about what happens after you die?"

- "Given that your time is limited, what legacy do you want to leave your family?"
- "What do you want your children and grandchildren to remember about you?"

If patients can no longer respond, the physician may ask the family, "How could we honor your father in his last phase of life?"

When Should Physicians Discuss Palliative Care with Patients?

Case 1-1 illustrated how physicians have a window of opportunity to discuss palliative care when the prognosis becomes limited, when the patient's suffering seems great, when therapies are ineffective or very burdensome, or when disease has progressed despite curative treatment. The following section will address whether such discussions are also useful earlier in the course of the disease.

Discussions Early in Serious, Progressive Chronic Illness

Palliative care is commonly considered terminal care, separate from and mutually exclusive of treatments that cure the underlying disease or treat the underlying pathophysiology (7). In this view, there is a sharp transition from chemotherapy to palliative care. Hospice care, the most familiar example of palliative care in the United States, is often considered only in the final stage of disease. This view stems largely from how hospice care has historically developed as a Medicare benefit. Under Medicare, physicians must certify that patients are expected to survive less than 6 months (1). The requirement of less than 6 months survival, together with inherent uncertainties in prognostication, may lead physicians to refer patients to hospice care late in their disease. The average patient enters hospice care only 1 month before death, and 16% enter only 1 week before death (12). Psychologically, hospice care requires that patients accept a limited prognosis and perhaps "give up" treatment for their underlying disease. However, many patients who would benefit from palliative care are unwilling to do so.

The common view that palliative care is separate from curative care or disease-oriented care needs to be rejected (1,7). Discussing palliative care only when patients have a poor prognosis has several serious drawbacks. Opportunities to relieve symptoms and achieve meaningful closure to life may be limited in the final weeks of life. Furthermore, patients may incorrectly infer that relieving symptoms is important only near the end of life or when life-sustaining interventions will be limited. Another problem is deciding what level of prognosis should trigger a discussion about palliative care. Currently, many doctors discuss palliative care when patients are expected to die in the very near future. However, it is difficult to identify such persons, particularly in diseases other than cancer. For instance, patients with congestive heart failure typically die from sudden arrhythmia and do not have a predictable terminal phase of steady decline. On the day before death, the average heart failure patient has a 50% likelihood of surviving 2 months (13). Thus, discussing palliative care only with patients who are expected to die soon will miss many patients who have a poor prognosis.

Physicians should take a "both/and" approach to palliative and disease-oriented care, rather than an "either/or" approach. Relieving distress, promoting quality of life, and attending to the psychosocial aspects of illness are always appropriate goals of care. When cancer patients undergo curative treatment, the side effects of chemotherapy need to be relieved, and psychosocial issues of coping with disease and treatment should be addressed. Patients with cancer may have considerable pain even early in their disease, yet physicians often hold back opioids at that time (14).

Early in disease, the goal of living longer is often added to palliative care. Discussions about palliative care can be put into the context of exploring patient and family concerns about the future, helping the patient be in control of care, and establishing shared goals for care. Routinely discussing palliative care early in the patient's course will assuage concerns that palliative care means that the physician is giving up or that the prognosis is worse than the physician has explicitly indicated. However, such discussions may seem problematic because patients and physicians alike may prefer to focus on hopes for cure and be reluctant to acknowledge suffering, fear, or death. Improved communication skills can help physicians in these discussions.

Discussions That Follow the Patient's Lead

Some patients question the usefulness of disease-oriented therapies, or talk about the burdens of illness, or express a wish to die. Physicians can explore why these issues have emerged at that time, discuss palliative care as an option, and commit to care for the patient and family throughout the illness if that is realistic (15). Follow the patient's lead. If a patient remarks, "I sometimes wonder if it's worth going on," we can respond by saying, "It sounds as if you've been having some fairly serious thoughts. Can you tell me more about what's on your mind?" This response communicates that the patient's concerns are taken seriously and invites clarification.

Despite the importance of responding openly to patients' questions and concerns, the approach of waiting for patients to take the lead in discussing palliative care has several disadvantages. It reinforces the perception that these discussions imply that the patient is dying. Also, we may miss cues that patients are ready to discuss such issues (6).

How Can Physicians Respond to Difficult Patient Statements and Questions?

Some patient answers to open-ended questions are disturbing or difficult to respond to. Suppose that in Case 1-1 the patient with refractory metastatic colon cancer said that the most important thing for him was to be at his daughter's birthday, almost a year away. How might the physician respond? Silence, when the physician is expected to agree, may convey the lack of agreement with the patient's statement. Subsequently, a response might be, "I can't even imagine how frightening it is to think about not being with her. You love her so much." This empathetic statement validates the patient's underlying emotion and encourages further discussion, without giving false hope. An alternative might be, "I know that you're trying very hard to keep your hopes up. Are you sometimes afraid that you won't be there for your family?" In this way, the physician can align with the patient's wish, without reinforcing unrealistic plans. Later, a more direct comment might be, " I know that you love your family and want to be there for them. How do you think you can best be there for them in the future?" This question might lead to a discussion of how financial planning is a way of taking care of loved ones.

In other cases, doctors may uncover problems we cannot fix. Some patients may no longer find meaning in life. Their families may be overwhelmed trying to cope with their illness. They may fear that they will be punished in the afterlife. When patients reveal such concerns, we may feel that we have made the situation worse, that we have failed, or that we are beyond our expertise. In these difficult situations, we can keep in mind several points. First, doctors have these feelings because we want to help patients and want to protect them. If we feel these goals are not being achieved, we may experience strong reactions. Second, our own feelings are often an important clue to how the patient is feeling. Thus, if we feel overwhelmed, frustrated, discouraged, or angry, the patient may have similar feelings. Third, we can clarify our role and self-expectations. Physicians usually cannot alter patients' fears of becoming a burden or being punished in the afterlife. Our attempts at reassurance may sound hollow. Yet even when problems are insoluble, the act of listening to the patient often is therapeutic. Patients are no longer alone with their problems if they believe that their concerns have been heard. Fourth, asking about the problems does not create them. Doctors need not make problems worse by talking with patients about them. Fifth, dying patients raise personal issues for physicians that stem from our own backgrounds and concerns. Finding a safe place to explore emotional reactions to dying patients is important for our own well-being and professional development. Finally, physicians do not have sole responsibility for responding to the patient's suffering. Nurses, social workers, chaplains, and psychiatrists can play helpful roles as well (10,16,17).

Although the issues are complex, some simple responses by physicians usually work. Instead of trying to fix problems, use the open-ended questions: "That sounds very distressing. Can you tell me more?" Although one instinct may be to end the conversation, it is more helpful to draw the patient out. By listening attentively, we communicate caring and commitment. Empathetic comments are also useful. By identifying the patient's emotions, we validate them and show the patient that he or she has been understood. Physicians should recall that the word "compassion" comes from the Latin words for "feel with" or "suffer with" the patient. Allying with the patient's hopes and wishes can also be soothing: "I wish that medicine had better answers."

Table 1-1 gives further suggestions on how to respond to difficult questions from patients about palliative care.

Table 1-1.   Difficult Patient Questions and Potential Physician Responses.

Patient Questions	Comments	Physician Responses
"How long do I have to live?"	"I wonder if it is frightening not knowing what will happen next or when (3)."	Acknowledging uncertainty can help ease its pain. An empathetic statement is useful before giving an estimate of prognosis.
	"Nobody knows for sure, but the average is 3 to 6 months. There are always exceptions, so it may be considerably longer, and it could be shorter."	A range allows the patient to make plans, while leaving room for exceptions.
"Does this mean that you are giving up on me?"	"Absolutely not, and I will explain in a minute. But first can you tell me what you mean by 'giving up'?"	Patients have different concerns about "giving up." Open-ended questions elicit the patient's specific concerns, which the physician can then address.
	"Nothing could be further from the truth. We are going to put more of our energy into relieving your suffering and improving your quality of life. We are going to work together to make the most of the time you have left."	Patients and families need to be reassured that they will not be abandoned if they give up curative treatment.
"Does this mean that she's about to die?"	"If I were thinking about my mother's death, I would feel very scared." After a pause to allow the patient to respond, the physician could continue, "We can't know exactly when she will die, but it could be soon. Are there things you would want to say to her if her death were to occur soon?"	Empathetic statements can lead to further exploration of the family member's feelings, a chance to support those feelings, and shared goals of care.
"Are you telling me that I am going to die?"	"No one can know for sure when that will happen, but it is possible in the near future. I am also asking you to think about how you would want to spend your time if it were limited."	An honest answer leaves hope and allows the patient to make realistic plans. Framing questions such as "What if time were limited?" are helpful.
What about experimental therapy? Should I go to the University Hospital?	"I can't even imagine how scary it may feel to have no control over this illness" (3).	Acknowledging the patient's emotions and their underlying cause helps prevent disagreements over "futile" interventions.
	"I wish we had better treatments for your disease. Let's look into it. Unfortunately, experimental therapy is unlikely to work and may add to suffering. I think you may be better off spending your time at home with your family, but let's see what choices are available."	The physician should help the patient explore all possibilities, but should make a clear recommendation. The decisions, of course, are the patient's.

How Can Physicians Discuss Palliative Care While Disease-Remitting Treatments Are Continued?

Discussing palliative care with patients is useful throughout the course of serious, progressive chronic illness, because the patient's condition, needs, and concerns may change. At each visit, routinely ask several open-ended questions to determine the patient's needs and suffering: "What concerns you most about your illness?" "How is treatment going for you and your family?" "Are you having discomfort or suffering that bothers you or limits what you do?" The next section suggests how to discuss integrating palliative care with disease-oriented treatment.

Continue Disease-Oriented Treatment While Providing Palliative Care

CASE 1-2. ELDERLY PATIENT WITH CARDIAC DISEASE AND LONELINESS

An 82-year-old woman had diabetes, azotemia, angina, and congestive heart failure. Her two daughters lived in the same building and did her housework and shopping. The patient was hospitalized for the third time in 2 months because of angina and an exacerbation of congestive heart failure.

At a family meeting, her primary physician asked, "Are you having any discomfort or distress?" The patient said she felt tired during the day and worried when her daughters were at work. When the doctor asked, "What concerns you the most about your condition?" the patient said that she wasn't afraid to die but hated feeling as though she could not breathe. She also said she didn't want to become a burden to her daughters. The doctor responded that there were many ways to relieve shortness of breath. Her daughters replied, "Don't be silly. You're not a burden. We'll do whatever it takes to keep you out of a nursing home." Further discussions revealed that the patient felt lonely and afraid when she was alone but would not ask her daughters to stay with her during the day. The patient and doctor decided on angiography and possible angioplasty or stenting in order to relieve ischemia-related shortness of breath. In addition, the family would look into geriatric day care.

In Case 1-2, the physician not only addressed biotechnical issues regarding congestive heart failure but also addressed the impact of the illness on the patient and her family. Although the family was loving and dedicated, the patient was afraid during the day when her daughters were at work. The plan for care combined an invasive, high-technology intervention, reassurance about future suffering, and a social intervention to improve the patient's current quality of life.

Increase Emphasis on Palliative Care While Maintaining Some Disease-Oriented Treatment

As disease progresses, palliative care may be given greater emphasis.

Refusal of Life-Sustaining Interventions

Angiography showed severe diffuse multivessel disease with poor distal runoff, which precluded revascularization. After explaining the results and their implications for further care, the physician asked, "What are your concerns about your illness?" The patient said she was afraid that things were going to get worse and worse. The doctor then asked, "What particular things frighten you the most?" The patient responded, "I don't want to spend my last days in the hospital. I've been in the hospital more in the past few months than in my first 80 years."

As physicians, we naturally want to reassure patients. However, offering reassurance before understanding patients' fears and concerns may seem premature or hollow. Thus, it is useful to ask additional open-ended questions when patients voice their concerns.

After further discussion, the patient decided against further hospitalizations, even though exacerbations could likely be reversed. "If my time has come, I'm ready. There's no point in dragging things out." Active treatment with diuretics, calcium channel blockers, nitrates, and aspirin was continued. She was referred to hospice care. Arrangements were made for home oxygen and administration of morphine if severe short-ness of breath or chest pain developed. One daughter had reservations about this plan, because she did not want to "give up." When asked, "What does 'giving up' mean to you?" she replied that her mother seemed comfortable and happy, except when her heart failure worsened. The physician said, "We will continue to treat her heart disease short of going to the hospital. We can't control how long she lives, but let's help her to make the best of the time she has."

When the doctor asked, "What might be left undone if you were to die today?" the patient replied that she regretted a falling out with her sister. The daughters, nurses, social worker, and physician talked with the patient about her relationship with her sister and encouraged her to call her sister or allow others to call.

Case 1-2 illustrates how palliative care can become more prominent as illness progresses. Active treatment for some medical problems can be continued while more attention is given to symptomatic relief. In addition to making plans for her medical problems, palliative care can include addressing the daughter's concerns and trying to help the patient reconcile with her sister. The daughter who didn't want to "give up" was able to refocus her energy into urging her mother to talk with her sister.

Address Misconceptions About Palliative Care

Physicians need to elicit and address misconceptions by patients and families about palliative care. One widespread misconception is that palliative care precludes high-technology interventions near the end of life.

CASE 1-3. INCORPORATING HIGH-TECHNOLOGY INTERVENTIONS INTO PALLIATIVE CARE

Two years after resection of a squamous cell carcinoma of the lung, a 64-year-old man developed brain metastases and received brain radiation therapy. He and his physician agreed that the goal was palliation, the treatments to include opioids, steroids, and a DNR order. He discussed his death with his physician. He developed ataxia and worsening headaches. A CT scan showed a recurrent brain metastasis. Because the patient already had received maximal radiation therapy, he was offered and chose to have neurosurgery. Before surgery, he stated that he did not want prolonged ICU care if complications developed. After resection of his brain lesion, his pain and ataxia decreased for several months.

Case 1-3 shows that appropriate palliative care may require high-technology interventions such as CT scans and invasive procedures such as neurosurgery. Palliative care should not be equated with low-technology care at home.

Other common misconceptions concern the use of opioids. The physician might ask, "What have you heard about morphine to relieve pain or shortness of breath?" Common misconceptions are that opioids are dangerous, cause addiction, shorten life, or are used only as a last resort. In fact, they are relatively safe, rarely if ever cause addiction in the terminally ill, and are a mainstay of therapy (18).

Still another misconception is that discussions about palliative care take too much time for busy physicians. These discussions can occur in small bits over time, and many good discussions take less than 10 min (19). Time spent on discussions may save more time later in the illness if misunderstandings, unrealistic expectations, or unaddressed concerns persist. Some evidence of the recognition of the importance of such discussions is seen in the new Medicare evaluation and management billing code for counseling time.

There may be objections to the approach of this chapter to the effect that open-ended questions and empathetic comments leave the physician too distant from the patient. Some may suggest that physicians share with patients their own thoughts on death and spirituality or anecdotes from their own experience. Although the intention to humanize care at the end of life is laudable, we believe that the focus should be on patients and their situation. Some patients may feel that someone who is not experiencing a terminal illness cannot understand their situation or give meaningful advice. Patients may not regard anecdotes about others as relevant to their situation. We should not underestimate the comfort patients experience when their concerns and needs are listened to and their feelings are accurately identified.

In our multicultural society, patients may have different attitudes towards discussing palliative care. In particular, some patients believe that discussion of death hastens death (20,21). However, the approaches recommended here, which encourage the physician to listen and allow the patient's concerns to drive the discussion, ensure respect for patient values.

Summary

Palliative care is important throughout the course of serious chronic illness. Sensitive interviewing techniques such as the use of open-ended questions and empathetic statements are helpful when discussing palliative care. Physicians can practice, experiment, and incorporate new interviewing skills into their practices. Continuing education programs that include role-playing or videotaping may be useful in developing such interviewing skills. In addition to addressing physical suffering, physicians can extend their caring by exploring and responding to psychosocial, existential, or spiritual suffering. Even though we cannot alleviate some types of suffering, active listening and empathy have therapeutic value.

REFERENCES

1. **Field MJ, Cassel CK, Eds.** Approaching Death: Improving Care at the End of Life. Washington, DC: National Academy Press; 1997.
2. **Lipkin M, Putnam SM, Lazare A, Eds.** The Medical Interview. New York: Springer Verlag; 1995.
3. **Buckman R.** How To Break Bad News. Baltimore: Johns Hopkins University Press; 1992:98-171.
4. **Doyle D.** Domiciary palliative care. In: Doyle D, Hanks GWC, MacDonald N, Eds. Oxford Textbook of Palliative Medicine, 2nd ed. New York: Oxford University Press; 1998: 957-73.
5. **Lipkin M, Frankel RM, Beckman HB, et al.** Performing the interview. In: Lipkin M, Putnam SM, Lazare A, Eds. The Medical Interview. New York: Springer Verlag; 1995:65-82.
6. **Tulsky JA, Chesney MA, Lo B.** How do medical residents discuss resuscitation with patients? J Gen Intern Med. 1995;10:436-42.
7. **Billings JA.** What is palliative care? J Palliative Med. In press.
8. **Foley K.** Pain assessment and cancer pain syndromes. In: Doyle D, Hanks GWC, MacDonald N, Eds. Oxford Textbook of Palliative Medicine, 2nd ed. New York: Oxford University Press; 1998:310-30.

9. **Chochinov HM, Wilson KG, Enns M, Lander S.** "Are you depressed?" Screening for depression in the terminally ill. Am J Psychiatry. 1997;154:674-6.
10. **Speck P.** Spiritual issues in palliative care. In: Doyle D, Hanks GWC, MacDonald N, Eds. Oxford Textbook of Palliative Medicine, 2nd ed. New York: Oxford University Press; 1998:805-14.
11. **Nathan Cummings Foundation and Fetzer Institute.** Spiritual Beliefs and the Dying Process: A Report on a National Survey. New York; October 1997.
12. **Christakis NA.** Timing of referral of terminally ill patients to an outpatient hospice. J Gen Intern Med. 1994;9:314-20.
13. **Lynn J.** An 88-year-old woman facing the end of life. JAMA. 1997;227:1633-40.
14. **Cleeland CS, Gonin R, Hatfield AK, et al.** Pain and its treatment in outpatients with metastatic cancer. N Engl J Med. 1994;330:592-6.
15. **Quill TE, Cassel CK.** Nonabandonment: a central obligation for physicians. Ann Intern Med. 1995;122:368-74.
16. **Monroe B.** Social work aspects of palliative care. In: Doyle D, Hanks GWC, MacDonald N, Eds. Oxford Textbook of Palliative Medicine, 2nd ed. New York: Oxford University Press; 1998:867-82.
17. **Breitbart W, Chochinov HM.** Psychiatric aspects of palliative care. In: Doyle D, Hanks GWC, MacDonald N, Eds. Oxford Textbook of Palliative Medicine, 2nd ed. New York: Oxford University Press; 1998:933-56.
18. **Levy MH.** Pharmacologic treatment of cancer pain. N Engl J Med. 1996;335:1124-32.
19. **Fischer GS, Tulsky JA, Rose MR, Arnold RM.** Opening the black box: an anlysis of outpatient discussions about advance directives. J Gen Intern Med. 1996;11(Suppl 1):115.
20. **Blackhall LJ, Murphy ST, Frank G, et al.** Ethnicity and attitudes toward patient autonomy. JAMA. 1995;274:820-5.
21. **Carrese JA, Rhodes LA.** Western bioethics on the Navajo reservation. JAMA. 1995;274:826-9.

CHAPTER 2

A Consensus-Based Approach to Practicing Palliative Care for Patients Who Lack Decision-Making Capacity

JASON H. T. KARLAWISH, MD • TIMOTHY E. QUILL, MD •
DIANE E. MEIER, MD

> *"As we grow older the world becomes stranger, the pattern more complicated of dead and living."*
>
> T.S. Eliot, "East Coker"

CASE 2-1. A WOMAN WITH SEVERE ALZHEIMER'S DISEASE

Mrs. Brown is a 73-year-old married woman with severe Alzheimer's disease. She is a retired schoolteacher and the mother of one daughter. For the past 3 years she has lived in a nursing home. Mrs. Brown requires assistance with all of the basic activities of daily living. Mr. Brown visits her daily and feeds her lunch. In the last several weeks, she has taken longer to finish small portions and, at times, she coughs while being fed. One morning, several hours after breakfast, Mrs. Brown developed agitation, a cough, and a temperature of 100.3°F.

A primary goal of palliative care is to relieve a patient's suffering in order to maximize the patient's dignity and quality of life (1). Respect for autonomous patient choice is part of the foundation of Western bioethics, but a patient with severe dementia typically cannot decide whether to receive predominantly palliative care or to continue potentially life-prolonging therapy. Others, such as family and care-givers, must choose for the patient. These decision-makers' goals and values may conflict with one another and potentially with those of the patient who now lacks the capacity to participate in the decision.

Conflicts are especially likely in decision-making about two common clinical problems: aspiration pneumonia and neurogenic dysphagia. These problems engage deep values about feeding, starvation, and the meaning of care for a patient with severe dementia (2). Furthermore, a patient's residence in a nursing home introduces additional problems related to regulations governing the management of a patient's weight loss and nutrition (3). How can a physician address these problems in a manner that serves the patient and achieves consensus among decision-makers? This case study presents an approach to creating a palliative care plan for patients with severe dementia.

The physician and director of nursing meet with Mr. Brown and the daughter. The physician explains the likely diagnoses of aspiration pneumonia and delirium and that, in the severe stages of dementia, aspiration pneumonia is a common problem caused by irreversible and progressive loss of the ability to chew and swallow food. Mr. Brown agrees that his wife has had trouble eating, and he describes how on some days she eats very little of even her favorite foods.

To prompt the family to tell more about their perception of how Mrs. Brown has changed, the physician asks, "I have only known Mrs. Brown for the last few months. Can you tell me how she was in the past, such as in the year before she came here?"

After hearing about Mrs. Brown's progressive loss of function, the physician says, "I think I have a better feel about how things have changed over the past few years. You know that Mrs. Brown has an incurable, progressive, and ultimately fatal disease. I can't say for sure when she'll die of her Alzheimer's disease, but, given its severity, we shouldn't be surprised when she does. Even if she does recover from this pneumonia, she will not recover her swallowing function. Recognizing this, we ought to care for her in a way that makes us confident that, after she's gone, we can say she was treated with dignity and respect.

"We must first decide how to treat her pneumonia. The options range from treating the discomfort of pneumonia but providing no antibiotics, to providing antibiotics in the nursing home or the hospital but not providing other invasive treatments, to hospitalization with the availability of life supports

including breathing machines if needed. No matter what is decided, we'll do our best to relieve any suffering she may have.

"I use two principles to help make these decisions. First, we must consider the patient's preferences. What is your understanding of what Mrs. Brown would want if she could tell us? Second, we should balance the burdens and benefits of each option in order to relieve her suffering and maximize her dignity and quality of life."

Table 2-1 summarizes the steps of the foregoing narrative. The physician's first step was to identify potential decision-makers. If Mrs. Brown had completed an advance directive that included a durable power of attorney for health care, that person would represent her in decision-making. However, most patients in nursing homes do not have advance directives (4), and even when they do the contribution of others such as family and formal caregivers can greatly assist the designated surrogate in decision-making (5,6). The physician can turn to close family members and others who know the patient well with the assurance that, even without an advance directive, the family's standing is established by case and statutory law (7). Except in cases where the patient has no family or has a family that acts in a manner that violates the patient's best interests, the physician is under no moral or legal authority to seek a guardian (7,8).

After identifying the decision-makers and clarifying Mrs. Brown's diagnoses, the physician's next step was to encourage Mr. Brown and his daughter to describe the course of Mrs. Brown's dementia. To do this, the physician asked them to describe how Mrs. Brown has changed. The purpose of this was to achieve a consensus among decision-makers about the patient's current disease state, prognosis, quality of life, and previously stated values (5). This sharing of narratives may expose important differences in beliefs and understandings in any of these domains that must be reconciled before consensus-based decision-making can proceed. Furthermore, it allows the physician to learn about the relationships between decision-makers and the patient, and between the decision-makers themselves. The more the physician understands these various understandings and relationships, the more likely he is to develop a plan that will respect Mrs. Brown as a person.

Next, the physician begins a discussion of palliative care. This requires conveying two points: a qualitative understanding of the

Table 2-1. How to Plan Palliative Care for Patients Who Lack Decision-Making Capacity.

An advance directive, if available, can provide guidance, but should not pre-empt conversation.

- Structure the decision-making as a process that is grounded in dialogue.

- The goal of this dialogue is to achieve consensus upon the meaning of emotionally charged terms like "suffering," "quality of life," "feeding" and "dying." This allows the family to come to terms with the meaning of the life and chronic illness of their loved one.

Recognize and acknowledge that this dialogue is often ambiguous because

- The decision-makers have a spectrum of views that may be held strongly or ambivalently.

- Terms like "suffering," "quality of life," "dignity," "feeding," "starving," and "dying" are subject to a variety of meanings and understandings.

The steps in this dialogue are

- Identifying the main participants in the decision-making process.

- Allowing the participants to narrate how the patient has come to this stage of his or her illness (e.g., "Can you tell me how your mother got to this point?").

- Teaching the decision-makers about the expected clinical course of the patient's disease (e.g., "Your wife has an incurable, progressive, and ultimately fatal disease. I can't say for sure when she'll die of her Alzheimer's disease, but, given its severity, we shouldn't be surprised when she does").

- Advocating for the patient's quality of life and dignity (e.g., "We ought to care for her in a way that makes us confident that after she's gone, we can say she was treated with dignity and respect").

- Providing guidance based on existing data and clinical experience.

- Avoiding claims of futility as a means to justify or reject a choice.

If conflict occurs:

- Understand and separate goals of medical care, clinical problems, and treatment choices from each person's perspective.

- Invent new solutions (e.g., a time-limited trial rather than an all-or-none solution).

- Avoid power struggles or personalizing the conflict.

- Call in a third party (e.g., clergyman, ethics or palliative care consultant).

- Do not violate fundamental values of the patient, family, or physician.

patient's prognosis and the general goal of palliative care. These points are made with the statement: "Mrs. Brown has an incurable, progressive, and ultimately fatal disease. I can't say for sure when she'll die of her Alzheimer's disease, but given its severity, we shouldn't be surprised when she does. We ought to care for her in a way that makes us confident that after she's gone, we can say that she was treated with dignity and respect." Although this physician believes strongly in palliative care for patients with severe Alzheimer's disease, he must respect that others may value an approach that equates survival with quality of life, and where available medical technology must always be used to prolong life.

Finally, the physician gave the family guidance on standards for decision making. He advised them to consider what is known of the patient's wishes and preferences given her current condition, such as potentially relevant statements that the patient made when competent in a living will, and he suggested that the family balance burdens and benefits in light of Mrs. Brown's current and potential future quality of life. These standards are explored together, not sequentially, because a patient's preferences for care under his current circumstances are based upon extrapolation from past situations or statements. Deciding how to care for Mrs. Brown using a rigid understanding of her past preferences fails to respect her present circumstances (9). Quality of life, while subjective and personal, incorporates these circumstances into what is known about her preferences and values, as well as those of her immediate family.

Missing from these instructions and recommendations to the family is an appeal to futility as grounds for decision-making. Futility refers to the claim that no desirable goal can be achieved by potentially life-prolonging treatment. Physicians frequently cite futility as a reason for recommendations to terminate further treatment (10). "Futility" is often portrayed as an objective term, but it can convey a negative judgment about a patient's quality of life or an informal cost-benefit analysis of an intervention, without explicitly engaging in a discussion of these issues from the differing perspectives of doctors and families. Furthermore, the term connotes that nothing more can be done for a patient, or that further intervention would be meaningless, or that life is of no current value. "Futility" frequently obscures an honest discussion of how people understand and value the patient's quality of life and the range of possibilities for palliative and life-prolonging interventions.

The husband and daughter agree that Mrs. Brown never expressed clear preferences about how she should be treated under her current clinical circumstances. "That's okay," the physician says. "We can still work together on a plan. Treatment in an acute hospital has burdens such as a change in environment and staff, and invasive and potentially uncomfortable treatments such as intravenous lines and blood tests. These need to be balanced against the potential benefits such as the increased chance of survival that might come from closer monitoring and more aggressive treatment. Antibiotics also have potential benefits and burdens. They will increase the chance that Mrs. Brown will survive, but she may survive in a more diminished condition. A helpful way to think through these choices is to come to some consensus upon her current quality of life and then decide what options will best preserve it."

In the ensuing discussion, Mrs. Brown's daughter, the physician, and the nurse feel that Mrs. Brown's quality of life is poor because she cannot communicate or move around, but the husband believes that she still enjoys his visits and being fed food he brings in from home. The daughter feels strongly that her mother would not want to live the way she is, but the husband disagrees. They all agree that if her quality of life deteriorates any further, even antibiotics would be too invasive.

The physician proposes a plan. "Mr. Brown, your visits are important. Let's work from that. I recommend that we keep her here at the nursing home where you can visit her as much as possible, provide antibiotics, and reassess her daily. If she deteriorates rapidly, our focus will shift exclusively to relieving her symptoms and minimizing her immediate suffering. I do not recommend providing CPR if she were to have a cardiac arrest or admitting her to the hospital."

The family agrees that the plan strikes a proper balance between benefits and burdens, giving Mrs. Brown a chance of recovery without subjecting her to a foreign environment or overly harsh treatments.

This decision-making process exposed two common features of caring for patients with severe dementia. First, clear information about the patient's wishes is typically unavailable. Second, decision-makers often have differing assessments of the patient's preferences and quality of life (11). In this case, the daughter and physician thought Mrs. Brown had a poor quality of life and were concerned that hospitalization and even antibiotics might further decrease her quality of life. The husband disagreed. They all were genuinely trying to act in Mrs. Brown's best interests without clear information about her preferences. They achieved compromise with the decision to give Mrs. Brown a therapeutic trial of antibiotics at the nursing home.

The physician structured an open decision-making process. The features of this process have been outlined in Table 2-1. Each person was given time to give his or her perception of how Mrs. Brown reached her present condition, to provide individual insight, and to ask questions. This interactive decision-making process allows everyone an opportunity to express how he or she understands the patient. The dialogue is essential for achieving consensus on a course of action that is responsive to both past and present patient realities, as well as to the concerns and priorities of the family (5,6).

In this case, the physician accepts the husband's grounds for treatment of pneumonia not solely because the husband has the legal authority to decide, but because the husband's perception that his wife still enjoys his daily visits is plausible. The physician remains uncertain if the husband is representing his wife's interests or his own, but he believes that the consensus reached best accommodates Mrs. Brown's interests as understood by the family and the health care team.

The goal of this dialogue was not to provoke conflict, but to more fully appreciate the meaning of the decision for the patient and her family (5,12). This approach to decision-making is grounded in narrative theory that unifies the clinical and moral dimensions of medicine (13,14). Clinical medicine is grounded in a series of stories told and interpreted from a variety of perspectives. The physician usually interprets these stories, using the science of clinical medicine, to develop a diagnostic and therapeutic plan. These same stories can be used to understand the patient's values, goals, and meanings of illness, which should guide the personal and moral sides of the same process. Only after multiple dimensions are explored and understood should the physician and patient (or patient's family) proceed with medical decision-making. This theory is practiced from the beginning of this case when the physician prompts Mr. Brown, his daughter, and the head nurse to describe their perception of Mrs. Brown's current condition, as well as how she has changed during recent years. The physician also shares his own perceptions. These stories are replete with perceptions that will decisively shape the process of medical decision-making on Mrs. Brown's behalf.

There are limitations to this theory. Consensus occurs in the context of choices. However, in the care of patients who lack decision-making capacity because of severe dementia and who live in a nursing home, local customs, beliefs, and systems of care can limit reasonable choices. For example, long-term care regulations are often wrongly believed to require that all residents with neurogenic dysphagia receive artificial nutrition and hydration. Surrogate decision-making laws are often misinterpreted to require a legally designated guardian for non-competent patients who lack an advance directive (3). In truth, although state laws vary in the degree of proof required of surrogate decision-makers who decide to withhold such treatment, these beliefs are incompatible with the legal right of patients and their families to refuse any and all medical treatments, including artificial nutrition and hydration, and they undermine the process of consensus-based decision-making (3). In addition to these misperceptions about laws and regulations, both health care systems and local community practices powerfully influence choices and decisions. For example, in the same community, two otherwise quality nursing homes may have dramatically different rates of enteral feeding for patients with severe dementia. In the SUPPORT study (15), large national variations in the rates of dying at home correlated with regional bed availability, not with patient and family preferences.

An additional practical concern of a busy internist is that these dialogues take time. No empirical data compare the time requirements of this method with those of other decision-making strategies. But the investments in mutual understanding and trust building should ultimately improve decision-making, promote higher quality care, and prevent conflict as the patient's illness progresses. These outcomes may well save time in future decision-making.

> *"What happens if I feed her?" asks Mr. Brown. "Isn't she going to choke or get a worse pneumonia? Should we feed her by a tube or in the vein?" The nurse suggests they do a test to see if it is safe to feed Mrs. Brown by mouth. "That will tell us if she needs a tube."*

The physician and family face a decision that is common to patients with severe dementia: how to manage dysphagia caused by the progressive loss of cortico-bulbar neural function. Mr. Brown's questions describe a typical decision-making cascade. Oral feeding is thought to put the patient at risk of aspiration pneumonia, so oral feeding should be stopped; mechanical feeding, either intravenous or enteral, is started so the patient does not aspirate or starve.

The physician explains that a feeding tube will allow the delivery of adequate nutrition and hydration, but it may not improve the quality or length of Mrs. Brown's life or prevent further aspiration. He appeals to the family to recall how they made the decision to only care for Mrs. Brown's pneumonia. The key issue is Mrs. Brown's quality of life and the pleasure she receives from her husband's daily visits and the food that he gives her.

Mr. Brown is unsure whether he would want to give up feeding his wife, and whether she would want him to. Both he and the daughter are concerned that if they only feed Mrs. Brown by mouth, the size of the portions and time it takes Mrs. Brown to eat will mean that she will not get enough to eat. Finally, they worry that any kind of oral feeding could result in another pneumonia.

The physician's challenge is to teach the family about the palliative care possibilities for patients with neurogenic dysphagia caused by severe dementia who develop aspiration pneumonia, including 1) permanent artificial feeding, avoiding all oral intake because of the risk of aspiration; 2) temporary artificial feeding during acute illness, and then resumption of "natural" feeding upon recovery; and 3) continued natural feeding despite the risk of aspiration (2). An important point here is that the presence or absence of a feeding tube is not a *prima facie* determinant of the quality of palliative care for a patient with severe dementia. The critical issue for patients like Mrs. Brown, their families, and health care providers is which approach to feeding will best serve the clinical goal of maximizing the benefits and minimizing the burdens of care. Table 2-2 summarizes some of the potential benefits and burdens of feeding tube placement.

Will a swallowing study help? Data from a swallowing study must be evaluated in context. During the acute illness, such a study is

Table 2-2. Potential Benefits and Burdens of Enteral Feeding Patients with Dysphagia Caused by Dementia.

Potential Benefits	Potential Burdens
• Prolongation of the life of a patient who cannot orally feed	• Prolongation of life when quality of life is poor
• Continuous delivery of quantifiable amounts of nutrition and hydration	• Restraints to prevent patient mishandling tube
• Ease of staff time and effort to feed a person	• Increased emphasis on technology of care and decreased emphasis on human touch, taste, smell of food
• Reimbursement as a skilled nursing need	• Medicalizes the dying process (focuses on the technology of nutrition/hydration)
• Possible reduction of pressure ulcers*	• Increased volumes of stool and urine production
• Possible reduction of aspiration*	• Continued risk of aspiration of oral secretions and regurgitated gastric contents
• Possible lessening of hunger and thirst*	• Increased severity of pressure ulcers via increased volumes of urine and stool
• Possible maintenance of nutritional indices*	• Bloating, weight gain
	• Hemorrhage, infection (unusual)
	• Loss of intimacy and attention during feeding and dry mouth if oral feeding is proscribed

Data from References 16, 18, 20, and 21.
*No reliable data support these claims.

unlikely to be helpful for assessing long-term swallowing function. Even when the pneumonia has cleared, the validity and reliability of swallowing evaluations vary among operators and techniques (16). For patients with severe dementia, the timing of the test and the cooperation and understanding of the patient also contribute to this variability. Swallowing studies can help in patient management by determining that certain food consistencies are more likely than others to place a patient at risk for aspiration (17) but are unlikely to answer questions about how much risk of aspiration is acceptable given the quality-of-life issues associated with "natural" eating versus feeding tube.

What kind of oral feeding has Mrs. Brown received? Do the nurses' aides and her husband have the skill and time to feed Mrs. Brown by mouth so that her risk of aspiration is reduced? Is the food the proper consistency to reduce the risk? The apparent technical ease of enteral feeding and its reimbursement as a skilled nursing task can exert subtle pressure to advocate its use, especially when "natural" eating becomes more difficult and time-consuming. Until these issues are explored, enteral feeding can become a misdirected solution to a problem caused by limited resources.

Are the short-term and long-term goals of enteral feeding understood from the outset? If the short-term goal is to help Mrs. Brown survive her pneumonia by acutely maintaining hydration and nutrition while the antibiotics take effect, then a temporary feeding tube could be indicated. If she survives the pneumonia, the feeding tube would be discontinued, and she could resume the "natural" feeding that seemed to be so central to her quality of life. If the goal is to deliver adequate hydration and nutrition in the long term, then this warrants a careful analysis of benefits and burdens in light of her values and quality of life with and without the tube.

Quality-of-life considerations, despite their subjectivity, must be fully integrated into these decisions by those who care for the patient. Otherwise, the inevitable uncertainty about the patient's true wishes will mean that all potentially life-prolonging therapies must be used despite their effect on the patient's immediate suffering. The smell and taste of even small amounts of food, as well as the human contact and touch of the feeding process, have inherent human value that go well beyond hydration and nutrition. These natural human processes are essential elements of most palliative care plans. Although they may sometimes be circumvented in the short run in the interest of surviving an acute illness, they should be given up in the long run only when it is clear that the patient's values warrant it.

Compared with oral feeding, will enteral feeding reduce Mrs. Brown's risk of aspiration? Although a randomized comparison has not been reported, the available studies suggest that enteral feeding does not remove the risk of aspiration (16,18). As long as the patient produces oral secretions and the oropharyngeal-gastric connections remain patent, the patient with severe dementia who is enterally fed remains at risk of aspirating oral and regurgitated gastric contents.

Will Mrs. Brown "starve" if she does not receive adequate nutrition and hydration? This question turns upon the meaning of "starve." If "starve" means the subjective sensations of thirst and hunger, we simply do not know the answer to this question because Mrs. Brown cannot tell us. Comparative data exist from patients in advanced stages of terminal diseases such as cancer who can report symptoms. Once their tolerated oral needs (moisture, sips as tolerated) are met, and they receive mouth care, such patients generally do not experience symptoms of thirst and hunger (19). If a trained person orally feeds Mrs. Brown and keeps her mouth moist and clean, her hunger and thirst are probably being satiated, even as she gradually stops eating and drinking toward the end of life. Continuing to offer Mrs. Brown appropriate food and fluids, and respecting her lack of interest in food, means she is not feeling starved (2).

The more medicalized meaning of "starve" is in the context of achieving objective indices of "normal" nutrition such as weight, nitrogen balance, serum levels of albumin and total protein, and the absence of decubitus ulcers. The term "normal" is offset with quotes because we really do not know what are or should be the normal nutritional parameters of a person with severe Alzheimer's disease. Data suggest that enteral feeding of patients with severe Alzheimer's disease may not prevent weight loss or prevent the progression of pressure ulcers (20,21).

These different meanings of "starve" suggest there is a tradeoff between biomedical concerns addressed by a feeding tube (hydration and nutritional measures) and quality of life concerns addressed by "natural" feeding (taste, smell, and human touch). Each approach may have its place, depending on the benefits and burdens in light of the patient's goals, values, and clinical circumstances (2).

> *After reviewing these issues, the husband and daughter decide that he, the husband, will receive instructions from a speech therapist, and continue feeding his wife by hand. Mrs. Brown gradually recovers from the pneumonia after a several-week course that entails considerable physical distress (cough, respiratory distress, fever, and agitation) that is palliated with opioids, humidified oxygen, nebulizers, antipyretics, and low-dose antipsychotic agents.*
>
> *Several months pass, and Mrs. Brown is now unable to use a straw. Her intake of spoon-fed fluids and food is scant. Her husband worries she will die of starvation. He approaches the physician for advice about how to proceed.*

Alois Alzheimer's case report describes a 51-year-old woman at the end of life: "At the end, the patient was completely stuporous; she lay in her bed with her legs drawn up under her, and in spite of all precautions she acquired decubitus ulcers" (22). Contemporary medical experience unfortunately remains much the same.

Mrs. Brown's Alzheimer's disease has progressed to the point where she is unable to eat by mouth, a natural outcome of this chronic and progressive neurodegenerative disease. She can no longer experience the one activity that all agreed gave her some quality of life: feeding by her husband. Although enteral feeding might extend the quantity of biological life, her chronic and progressive neurodegenerative disease has progressed to the degree that she lacks most cortical functions (23).

Mrs. Brown's physician has consistently advocated a palliative approach as the standard of care for patients suffering from severe Alzheimer's disease and therefore explicitly advocates decision-making based upon a collective understanding of the patient's quality of life. This means revisiting the discussion with the family and staff caring for Mrs. Brown to achieve a consensus about what Mrs. Brown would tell them to do if she could understand her current circumstances, and what it would mean to use or not use a feeding tube. Understanding these perceptions and meanings are the foundation for a consensus about her subsequent medical care (24).

The physician, Mr. Brown, Mrs. Brown's daughter, and the nurse review Mrs. Brown's life and the recent events. After some discussion the physician says: "Her Alzheimers's disease has progressed to the point where she's dying. We ought to come up with a plan that minimizes her immediate suffering and maximizes the quality of her life."

A vigorous discussion follows. Eating was the one meaningful activity that remained in Mrs. Brown's life, but artificial feeding cannot serve the same function. Without that activity, the husband now believes that her quality of life is too poor to warrant the burdens of a feeding tube. A plan is agreed upon to provide comfort measures only. She will be offered tastes and smells of her favorite foods and drinks, mouth and skin hygiene, lots of human contact, including repositioning and massage, but no enteral or intravenous nutrition or hydration.

Seven days later Mrs. Brown dies.

Discussion

This case presents a number of common challenges to the practice of palliative care for patients with severe dementia. Mrs. Brown could not speak for herself and, like most Americans, she did not complete an advance directive. Even if she had, the preferences she expressed when competent may well have been indeterminate guides for managing her actual problems. In her present condition, she could not tell us if she was suffering or describe her quality of life, so the meaning of her signs and symptoms had to be interpreted. Furthermore, as a wife, mother, patient, and resident of a nursing home, she lived in a diverse community that had different views about what ought to be done for her. Finally, her problems included dementia complicated by aspiration pneumonia. No evidence supports that feeding via an enteral route will prevent this and other common complications of terminal dementia (16,18,20,21). Despite the lack of evidence regarding patient preferences and quality of life, beliefs about the meanings of care, starvation, and feeding and the need to provide loving care often motivate the pursuit of artificial nutrition and hydration.

This case illustrates a palliative care strategy for clinicians to address these challenges. This strategy is grounded in the theory that decisions for patients such as Mrs. Brown are the result of dialogue and consensus building. The physician's initial investment of time may serve to minimize the time and effort needed for future decisions. The physician's duty is to inform all participants that Mrs. Brown has a chronic, irreversible, and ultimately fatal disease but also to learn from them about Mrs. Brown's values and quality of life. Thus, decisions about hospitalization, antibiotics, and enteral nutritional support via a PEG tube are choices that ultimately shape the way she will live the last phase of her life. Accordingly, the physician consistently focuses on the patient's dignity and quality of life.

As a result of this dialogue, a family may decide that continued efforts to prolong life are critical regardless of the severity of the patient's disease. Physicians attempting to practice palliative care for patients with severe Alzheimer's disease may have difficulty working with such families' assessments of the benefits and burdens of treatment. Principles of negotiation are often useful to achieve consensus under these circumstances (see Table 2-1). Every effort should be made to find common ground. In general, the family's assessment and decision should be respected because, except in cases that clearly violate the best interests or previous wishes of the patient, the family has the final say in representing the patient in decision-making. Families have to live with themselves and their role in these decisions long after the patient has died. Furthermore, palliative care is not an "all or nothing" proposition. Careful relief of symptoms remains a basic standard of medical care, regardless of the use of coexisting life-prolonging treatments.

Conversely, some medical practitioners or long-term care institutions see their job as prolonging life because of religious principles, personal training, or misperceptions of the law. These practitioners or institutions should make their philosophy known from the outset, especially if they feel obligated to override the values and wishes of patients and families because they will be unable to pursue this consensus-based approach.

The meaning of suffering is personal and is a challenge to evaluate in patients with dementia. Even when suffering is recognized, its relief may be relegated to the pursuit of another goal, such as the preservation of life at all costs or hope for a miraculous cure. However, through the process of repeatedly listening to the perspectives of each participant and involving them in a consensus-based interaction, decisions that respect the patient's dignity and quality of life can generally be achieved.

REFERENCES

1. **Doyle D, Hanks G, MacDonald N.** Oxford Textbook of Palliative Care, 2nd ed. New York: Oxford University Press; 1998.
2. **Lo B, Dornbrand L.** Sounding board. Guiding the hand that feeds: caring for the demented elderly. N Engl J Med. 1984;311:402-4.
3. **Meisel A.** Barriers to forgoing nutrition and hydration in nursing homes. Am J Law Med. 1995;21:335-82.
4. **Janofsky JS, Rovner BW.** Prevalence of advance directives and guardianship in nursing home patients. J Geriatr Psychiatry Neurol. 1993;6:214-16.
5. **Kuczewski M.** Reconceiving the family: the process of consent in medical decisionmaking. Hastings Cent Rep. 1996;26:30-7.
6. **Brock D.** What is the moral authority of family members to act as surrogates for incompetent patients? Milbank Q. 1996;74:599-618.
7. **Meisel A.** The Right to Die. 2nd ed. New York: Wiley; 1996.
8. **Brock D, Buchanan A.** Deciding for Others: The Ethics of Surrogate Decision Making. Cambridge: Cambridge University Press; 1989.

9. **Dresser R.** Dworkin on dementia: elegant theory, questionable policy. Hastings Cent Rep. 1995;25:32-8.

10. **Prendergast T, Luce J.** Increasing incidence of withholding and withdrawal of life support from the critically ill. Am J Respir Crit Care Med. 1997;115:15-20.

11. **Sulmasy D, Terry P, Weisman C.** The accuracy of substituted judgements in patients with terminal diagnoses. Ann Intern Med. 1998;128:621-9.

12. **Quill T, Brody H.** Physician recommendations and patient autonomy: finding a balance between physician power and patient choice. Ann Intern Med. 1996;125:763-9.

13. **Bruner J.** Acts of Meaning. Cambridge, MA: Harvard University Press; 1990.

14. **Hunter K.** Doctor's Stories: The Narrative Structure of Medical Knowledge. Princeton, NJ: Princeton University Press; 1991.

15. **The SUPPORT Principal Investigators.** A controlled trial to improve care for seriously ill hospitalized patients. The Study to Understand Prognoses and Preferences for Outcomes and Risks of Treatments (SUPPORT). JAMA. 1995;274:1591-8.

16. **Ahronheim J.** Nutrition and hydration in the terminal patient. Clin Geriatr Med. 1996; 12:379-91.

17. **Curran J, Groher M.** Developmental and dissemination of an aspiration risk reduction diet. Dysphagia. 1990;5:6-12.

18. **Finucane TE, Bynum JPW.** Use of tube feeding to prevent aspiration penumonia. Lancet. 1996;348:1421-4.

19. **McCann R, Hall W, Groth-Juncker A.** Comfort care for terminally ill patients. JAMA. 1994;272:1263-6.

20. **Henderson C, Trumbore L, Mobarhan S, et al.** Prolonged tube feeding in long-term care: nutritional status and clinical outcomes. J Am Coll Nutr. 1992;11:309-25.

21. **Finucane TE.** Malnutrition, tube feeding and pressure sores: data are incomplete. J Am Geriatr Soc. 1995;43:447-51.

22. **Alzheimer A.** Uber eine eigenartige Erkangung der Hirnrinde. Allegemeine Zeitscher Psychiatr Psychisch-Gerichtliche Medizin. 1907;64:46-8 (English translation available in Arch Neurol. 1967;21:109-10).

23. **Walshe T, Leonard C.** Extensions of the syndrome to include chronic disorders. Arch Neurol. 1985;42:1045-7.

24. **Hurley A, Volicer L, Rempusheski V, Fry S.** Reaching consensus: the process of recommending treatment decision for Alzheimer's patients. Adv Nurs Sci. 1995;18:33-43.

CHAPTER 3

Respecting Cultural Differences at the End of Life

LAVERA M. CRAWLEY, MD • PATRICIA A. MARSHALL, MD •
BARBARA A. KOENIG, MD

The concept of a "good death" has been defined as being "free from avoidable distress and suffering for patients, families, and caregivers; in general accord with patients' and families' wishes; and reasonably consistent with clinical, cultural, and ethical standards" (1). First, we present three cases in which an important goal for each patient is care that improves the quality of the end-of-life experience. We will address issues that physicians need to consider and actions that physicians and patients can take together to reach the goal of a "good death."

CASE 3-1. A WOMAN WITH AIDS: DISCUSSIONS OF ADVANCE DIRECTIVES

W.M., a 49-year-old woman with AIDS, has been seen recently for new neurologic symptoms. Despite trials with various combinations of anti-retroviral drugs, she has begun to show signs of deterioration, including mental status changes. The issue of future decision-making in the event of incapacity was raised early in the course of her disease; at the time of that discussion, W.M. seemed to want everything done to help her survive if she were to become terminal. She declined, however, to execute an advance directive. The patient's daughter, who usually accompanied her mother to clinic appointments, adamantly agreed with this goal. Concerned with the recent change in W.M.'s health status, the provider again raised the issue of the patient's preferences for end-of-life care. This time the daughter expressed a strong desire that her mother not receive technological interventions ("no machines," in her words) during resuscitative efforts in the event of acute deterioration. The physician was unclear whether this represented a change in the patient's preference or was now a view held by the daughter alone. Given this confusion, how might the physician foster clearer communication regarding end-of-life preferences?

CASE 3-2. AN ELDERLY MAN WITH ADVANCED LUNG CANCER: DISCLOSING A DIAGNOSIS

P.C., a 77-year-old man, was brought to a local medical clinic by his adult son for back pain, fatigue, weight loss, and cough. In the course of his work-up, the patient's son asked that his father not be told the diagnosis and prognosis. This request conflicted with the physician's concerns for truth-telling, patient autonomy, informed consent, and the patient's right to information about care. When the work-up confirmed a diagnosis of inoperable adenocarcinoma of the lung with multiple metastases to bone, brain, and liver, the physician felt that she could not honor the son's request to withhold this information. The family insisted that the patient not be told, stating that such knowledge would create more harm than good. What strategies might be employed to assist with the ethical dilemma of conflicting values?

CASE 3-3. A MAN WITH ADVANCED PROSTATE CANCER: DISCUSSIONS OF MEDICAL FUTILITY

L.B., 59 years of age, was diagnosed with advanced metastatic prostate cancer. Early on he refused surgery but did undergo radiation treatment of his prostate and metastatic bone lesions. He lives with his wife and a large extended family. Although he stays at home, he has frequently required transfers to the hospital or to a skilled nursing facility for management of pain, nutritional needs, or other acute conditions. Throughout the course of his illness, he has angrily refused to discuss options such as hospice care and wants diagnostic and therapeutic interventions for his cancer and other chronic medical problems. He has a written advance directive indicating his desire for aggressive interventions should he require artificial measures to sustain his life. The physician in this case strongly suspects that this insistence on aggressive care may stem from the patient's failure to understand adequately the limits of medical technology. For those requests that are deemed medically futile, how might the physician discuss the goals of palliative care with the patient?

The definition of a good death implies the need for good communication to assist in such tasks as the disclosure of a terminal diagnosis or poor prognosis, and the eliciting of patient preferences in decision-making, including advance care planning. It also requires that attention be paid to psychosocial and spiritual concerns, ethical decision-making, and supportive palliative care, including adequate symptom control. It assumes that providers and patients, their families and proxies, have a shared understanding of what constitutes distress and suffering. It also assumes that clinical, cultural, and ethical standards are not in conflict.

Of note in each of the cases presented above is that, aside from gender, we have no indicators of the lived experiences, cultural influences, or social positions of these patient-factors that strongly influence end-of-life preferences. Below, when these cases are revisited, important cultural features will be included. What has been presented thus far in the standard medical narrative is strikingly one-dimensional. The patients are understood only through their clinical descriptions, told through a medical perspective that presumes that their problems are amenable to medical or medical ethics solutions. The cultural background features of these patients (which may give shape and meaning to their underlying explanatory models of health, illness, or death, and to the symbolic structures [e.g., language, ritu-als, roles] used in communicating and negotiating care) is hidden. Without this critical information, physicians are handicapped in pro-viding competent, sensitive, and effective end-of-life care to these patients.

Demographic transformations of American society will increase the likelihood of physicians encountering ethnic and cultural diversity in the clinical setting. Census estimates for 2000 show a continuing rise of Asian/Pacific Islander and Hispanic populations since the 1980 census. The same period shows an increase in all other ethnic groups except for non-Hispanic whites, whose population has decreased. Along with demographic transformations, a changed social climate now fosters the goal of multiculturalism. Attending to the needs of a culturally diverse population requires physicians to broaden the criteria used in defining a good death. For example, the meaning and outward expression of distress and suffering will vary across cultures, as do values inherent in the wishes of patients and their families.

To provide effective end-of-life care, physicians must attend to the variety of psychosocial and spiritual beliefs and the forms through which they are expressed. Similarly, physicians must respect the diversity of ethical values that support decision-making, even when these values do not match those of the provider or of the health care system (2).

Culturally Effective End-of-Life Care: Basic Concepts

Practicing culturally effective care can support the needs of both physi-cians and the patients they serve who are facing the end of life. Attention to basic concepts of cross-cultural medicine can help physi-cians negotiate the complexities of difference (Table 3-1).

Cultural Competence versus Cultural Sensitivity

Patient encounters involving cultural diversity highlight the need for caregivers to provide services that are culturally competent and that exhibit sensitivity to diverse communities. Medical schools and hospi-tals have implemented multicultural curricula aimed at teaching med-ical students and physicians how to deliver effective health care with-in an increasingly diverse American society. In these training models, as well as in the medical literature, such concepts as "cultural compe-

Table 3-1. Basic Concepts of Culturally Effective End-of Life Care.

Concept	Provider Requirements
Cultural competence	Knowledge base of cultural values, beliefs, and practices plus technical capacities (e.g., communication skills, use of interpreters, cultural etiquette)
Cultural sensitivity	Awareness of and respect for the role of culture in individual makeup
Culture of medicine	Awareness of the impact of explanatory models, values, and practices that privilege scientific evidence and individualism
Avoidance of stereotyping	Understanding the fluidity of cultural identity and allowing for individual behavior outside of cultural norms
Cross-cultural palliative care	Recognition of culturally mediated practices (e.g., outward expression of pain, beliefs regarding nutrition, dietary preferences) that affect symptom and pain management
Grief and bereavement	Recognition of varieties of mourning practices and observances related to care of the body after death

tence," "cultural sensitivity or humility," and "culturally effective health care," have been variously used without uniform agreement as to their meaning (3-8). These concepts can be divided into two categories of physician attributes: those that are skills-based (competence) and those dealing with attitudes or perspectives (sensitivity) (6,8).

As in the requirements for clinical competence—-solid knowledge base plus technical capacity—-cultural competency requires knowledge of the cultural and ethnic values, beliefs, and behaviors held by the patients from the cultures likely to be cared for. It also requires proficiency with technical capacities (such as communication skills) that allow the physician to take appropriate actions within a cross-cultural context. Cultural sensitivity, on the other hand, refers to the provider's awareness and respect for patients' cultural values, beliefs, and world views (4). An unfortunate feature of much cultural awareness training in the United States is the implicit assumption that culture is something that adheres to distant "others." The concept and goals of cultural sensitivity must be expanded to include provider awareness of the values and perspectives that they hold, from both their personal culture-of-origin and the biomedical worldview, a potent culture in its own right.

The Culture of Medicine

The fact that medicine itself is a cultural system is often hidden from our awareness. Those of us embedded within the biomedical system learn to assume the authority of science. These assumptions are substantiated by medicine's contribution to major advances in the control of disease and illness. Technological successes in medicine have not only contributed to the capacity to prolong life but have also made possible, paradoxically, some aspects of the process of dying. Death as a medical event has its own specific language, values, and practices that must be translated, interpreted, and negotiated with patients, families, and communities who are outside of the professional domain of medicine. Training in cultural competence and sensitivity should include the awareness of this dynamic.

Although the values held by medicine may privilege ethical notions of individual autonomy, disclosure, and informed choice, these values are not universally shared (9-14). For example, studies on how American ethnic populations value individual autonomy suggest that what constitutes self-determination for an identified patient may, in some populations, extend beyond an individual to include the family as a whole and the larger community (9). Consequently, it may be more culturally appropriate in some circumstances to negotiate the disclosure of diagnoses and treatments with members of a family first, rather than with the patient. Knowledge of culture-based beliefs and mores do not, in and of themselves, provide guidance on how to proceed when these values are at odds with the ethical framework of the physician, the larger medical system, or society.

Avoidance of Stereotyping

It is highly impractical to expect a medical provider to master the values, beliefs, and practices held by the vast numbers of ethnic populations and the myriad cultural and other important differences that exist within these groups. Cultural guidebooks that compile information for various ethnicities and countries can familiarize physicians with such culture-based variables as languages, religions, family roles, sick care, and death practices (15,16). Although these guidelines may be useful, it is important to recognize that neither culture nor cultural beliefs about end-of-life care can be easily represented or communicated. Factors such as gender, socioeconomic class, education, immigrant or refugee status, or religion interact with patients' cultural backgrounds in important ways, and cultural beliefs are not static and unchangeable. Simply learning about the cultural values of various ethnic groups runs the risk of stereotyping individuals "to create a 'shopping list' of cultural characteristics...in order to systematize and 'tidy up' culture in the same way as are other epidemiologic variables...." (17). Failure to appreciate the fluidity of cultural identity risks the misappropriation of values and behaviors.

Concepts of culture and ethnicity are useful for generalizing about population trends. However, they cannot predict individual behavior. They may be useful as markers for hypothesis testing, for adjusting the clinical index of suspicion or threshold for ordering tests, but not for limiting options in diagnosis or treatment. Stereotyping patients can be dangerous when behaviors of great significance, such as those at the end of life, are involved.

Cross-Cultural Palliative Care

The goals of palliative medicine are to control symptoms related to the suffering that may accompany the dying process (18-20). Barriers to these goals exist when providers fail to recognize the role that culture plays in the dying process. Many areas of palliative care involve culturally mediated practices, including pain control, feeding and nutrition, distress (both psychosocial and spiritual), and bereavement (21). Both cultural competence and sensitivity in dealing with patients in cross-cultural settings are needed if assessment and treatment efforts are to succeed. Symptom management in cross-cultural contexts requires adept attention to differences in the expression of pain and suffering and to the perceptions and customs related to the body (22,23). Studies showing that minority patients routinely receive inadequate analgesia, including palliative treatment for cancer-related pain, highlight the need for both cultural sensitivity and competence in this area (24-26).

Grief and Bereavement

Knowledge of the mourning practices of various ethnic groups can help providers with appropriate and timely intervention in the grieving process (23,27,28). Mourning practices may also include observance of cultural or religious rites involving the body during the dying process (such as prayers or blessings) or immediately after death (such as bathing or wrapping in ritual clothing). Physicians, social workers, nurses, and other members of the health care team can help families negotiate with hospital services to allow for personal rituals that do not otherwise compromise care. Those customs that may cause conflict or create hazards, such as the burning of incense, can be addressed respectfully and creative compromises sought that honor the intent of the practice. Understanding the importance of such rituals can support bereavement processes and end-of-life discussions about such topics as organ procurement and the performance of autopsies (29).

Culturally effective end-of-life care, necessary for facilitating a patient's and family's experience of a "good death," can result when the combined effects of technical competence and provider sensitivity interact in mutual partnership with patients, families, and communities. Technical competence should address such issues as improving communication, including working through language interpreters; addressing issues unique to immigration; and negotiating ethical conflicts. Attitudinal issues that should be addressed include problems with conflating culture with other demographic variables; the impact of implicit attitudes that may bias physicians against certain cultural practices or for values and practices reflecting the culture of medicine; and the avoidance of stereotyping patients.

Implications for End-of-Life Care

The cases introduced earlier in this paper will now be revisited with a fuller description of the cultural backgrounds and their influences on each case. Each case will address problems involved in end-of-life care, followed by potential strategies that may help providers give that care in a culturally effective manner (Table 3-2). The first two cases illustrate strategies for technical competence, and the third case identifies attitudinal perspectives that facilitate effective end-of-life care.

Table 3-2. Issues and Strategies for Culturally Effective Care.

Technical Issues	Provider Strategies
Communication: general concerns	1. Be alert for need for clarity, even when patients share same language or use local dialects 2. Ascertain if comprehension exists in both directions (physician↔patient)
Language barriers	3. Use trained medical interpreters 4. When possible, avoid using family or friends of patient as translators
Ambiguous social gestures	5. Increase awareness of social and cultural etiquette for specific populations
Caring for specific populations	6. Increase knowledge of the particular cultural, economic, sociopolitical, and historical contexts (available from guidebooks, community informants, religious leaders, or professional colleagues)
Conflicting values	7. Enhance communication 8. Elicit information regarding patient or family explanatory models and values; identify physician's values 9. Identify shared values and assess willingness to modify positions 10. Seek creative solutions that accommodate both sets of values 11. Seek consultation to assist in this process or when parties are not willing to modify positions
Attitudinal Issues	
Level of trust in the health care system	12. Respectfully inquire about past or present incidents that may have engendered mistrust 13. Identify possible behaviors by medical staff or physicians that were considered impolite or abusive 14. Apologize and assure patient that you will seek appropriate remedial actions if abuses were identified
Implicit negative attitudes	15. Providers should honestly examine negative attitudes they may implicitly hold toward certain populations and eliminate behaviors that may be discriminatory

Technical Aspects of Culturally Effective Care

Wilma Martinez is a 49-year-old immigrant from El Salvador who moved to this country to live with her eldest daughter. The physician who cared for Mrs. Martinez worked in a busy public health facility that served many non-English-speaking immigrants and refugees. Mrs. Martinez spoke only Spanish. Through her daughter's translations, Mrs. Martinez appeared to comprehend the details of her illness and treatment. When asked if she understood what the doctor was saying, she nodded yes.

During a clinic visit at which the daughter was unable to be present, the physician arranged for a Spanish interpreter. When the physician raised the issue of end-of-life preferences, the interpreter informed the physician that Mrs. Martinez thought the technological interventions used during resuscitation (such as ventilatory support or electrical shock) were devices that would actually hasten her death, thus her desire for "no machines."

Recognizing that language barriers had contributed to ineffective end-of-life communications, the provider arranged for trained interpreters to be present at all subsequent visits. All discussions were handled to ensure that both physician and patient understood perspectives held by the other. The provider asked both Mrs. Martinez and her daughter to share their understandings of the progression of her illness. In turn, he carefully explained all available options and potential outcomes. Because this provider cared for a large number of Latino patients, he also consulted the literature and community resources to increase his knowledge and understanding of the cultural, economic, sociopolitical, and historical contexts of this diverse community. Additionally, he inquired further into Mrs. Martinez' life story and used subsequent clinic visits as opportunities to add to his understanding of the role that her illness played in the larger context of her life.

Identified Problems

The problems encountered in this case of a Salvadoran woman with AIDS center around communication issues, primarily those related to language and cultural etiquette. Advance care planning discussions were initially hampered by the daughter's misinterpretation of technical information. This not only illustrates problems resulting from different languages (English versus Spanish); it also demonstrates how cultural misunderstandings can occur within the same language (medical versus lay usage of English). This case also illustrates the need to understand how the varied manifestations of social etiquette in language, touch, body language, and other critical meta-communications affect the doctor-patient relationship. Although Mrs. Martinez nodded affirmatively during discussions of advance directives, this gesture may have respresented a more complex meaning than simple agreement.

Mrs. Martinez' case also raises the issue of immigrant and refugee status. A patient's legal status will have a significant effect on health care access, compliance, and follow-up (30,31). Continuity of care, a critical factor in end-of-life care, may not be possible for the patient whose resident status is uncertain. Additionally, patients who have immigrated from countries that have experienced war or political violence, such as those from nations in Central America or Southeast Asia, may have been direct or indirect victims of political torture or trauma and could express mistrust and uncertainty in negotiations with health care systems and authorities, particularly when medical interventions involve physical touch (32). This mistrust, although potentially misplaced, is a legitimate and rational response, given a history of institutionally sanctioned trauma (33).

Strategies for Effective Care

Case 3-1 illustrates the need to understand challenges in communication when the patient and provider differ in language and culture. As tempting as it may be to rely on family members or other inexperienced translators, this should be avoided. Using family members may also violate privacy issues and generate conflicts around disclosure, both of which can create barriers to adequate information exchange.

Any language difference, even those that exist within the provider's own language (e.g., African-American vernacular English, youth slang), should send an alert for the need to seek greater clarity

(31). There can be no substitute for "effective, efficient, and reliable communication" between a provider and patient facilitated by trained medical interpreters (34). These interpreters provide more than mechanical translation of words. They negotiate and mediate across explanatory models of health and illness. They can also interpret culture-based gestures that may represent social etiquette. Their role in increasing the understanding of both parties (physician and patient) makes them highly influential in the communication process (30). A culturally competent provider must be aware of the complexities of such interchanges. In discussing complex subjects, such as delivering news of a bad prognosis, the physician and interpreter should plan their communication strategies in advance of the patient encounter. Although trained interpreters can help when language barriers exist, physicians must bear in mind that interpreters themselves may influence the content of messages conveyed during translations. Physicians should ascertain whether conceptual comprehension exists both with interpreters and with patients.

Providers who care for large numbers of patients from a specific population, as does the physician in the case of Mrs. Martinez, should increase their knowledge and understanding of that community. This information is available through guidebooks and other resources and might have helped the physician interpret the meaning of Mrs. Martinez's social gestures. Rather than indicating agreement, Mrs. Martinez's affirmative nod may have reflected cultural dynamics regarding authority or power or social expectations of politeness and respect rather than indicate agreement (35). It is critical in end-of-life discussions to be able to distinguish between responses that are merely polite and cordial, such as nodding or smiling, and those that reflect the patient's actual underlying feelings and desires.

Learning the larger narrative of the patient's culture, such as sociopolitical stories of Central American refugees who fled war and oppression, can help situate and contextualize the patient's narrative into the larger story of their community (30,32,33). This may require the cultivation of resources, such as religious leaders and community workers, to serve as part of an information network (36). These key informants can identify sensitive areas of communication and may offer insights that improve end-of-life interactions. Providers should attempt to ascertain the patient's life story, even if secondhand accounts from family or other providers are the only available sources.

CASE 3-2. AN ELDERLY KOREAN WITH ADVANCED LUNG CANCER: TRUTH-TELLING, DISCLOSURE, AND DIFFERENCES IN VALUES IN END-OF-LIFE DECISION-MAKING

Paul Choi is an elderly Korean-American who speaks English well. He was very active in Christian missionary work and often discussed this with his physician. Mr. Choi's Judeo-Christian beliefs in addition to the absence of a language barrier between Mr. Choi and the physician removed any question of need for translators or interpreters and supported the physician's assumption that direct communication with the patient was appropriate. The physician valued the idea of shared decision-making and believed that it was morally wrong to deny Mr. Choi the opportunity to participate fully in his care. During the discussion about disclosing diagnosis and prognosis, Mr. Choi's son was adamant that all communication was to go through him alone. The son considered failure to respect this request as tantamount to wishing harm to his father, an accusation that angered the physician. Sensing an impasse, the provider sought consultation.

The goal of the ethics consultation was to find a common ground for both the physician and the Choi family to participate in shared decision-making. This process of negotiation required not only ascertaining which values were operating for both the physician and the Choi family (which included Mr. Choi) but seeking an understanding of the intentions behind these values. The objective would then be to seek creative solutions that met the underlying goals for care. Following this strategy, the doctor explained her moral stance, based on the principle of autonomy or respect for persons, which undergirds the patient's right to make decisions. It was suggested that the physician next try to determine Mr. Choi's expectations of the doctor, as his primary provider, and of his family. Mr. Choi informed his physician that he preferred information to be given to his son, who was the spokesperson for the entire family, and who would be responsible for any decisions regarding his care.

Identified Problems

To spare his needless suffering, the Choi family wished to keep Mr. Choi from knowing the truth about his condition. In contrast, Mr. Choi's physician valued truth-telling and individual autonomy in the Western tradition of medical ethics and law. These values conflicted with those held by this Korean family. To them, the appropriate unit of decision-making was the family—not the individual patient—and it was the duty of the eldest son to serve both his father's and family's best interests by shielding Mr. Choi from the burdens of his disease (9). The values held by the son and by the physician seemed mutually exclusive, creating an initial impasse.

Strategies for Effective Care

Negotiating the myriad ethical choices facing the end of life (issues of disclosure of diagnosis or prognosis, decisions to limit treatment, the use of advance directives) requires an account of the values and beliefs that inform the explanatory models of life, health, illness, and death held by all involved parties. When patients, families, and providers share an understanding of and are in agreement with each other about the clinical, cultural, and ethical standards of medicine, the risk of conflicts regarding end-of-life decision-making are lessened. Moral conflicts arise when there is a clash regarding the underlying values, such as those between Mr. Choi's family and the physician.

Opportunities for such clashes may be avoided by enhancing communication among patients, families, and providers. In addition to issues noted in the first case presented—language, social etiquette, and the need to understand community history—ethical conflicts may require additional skills. To facilitate shared decision-making in cross-cultural situations, providers (and patients) must each assess their willingness to modify their position to seek creative solutions that include "both/and" versus "either/or" perspectives (10,37). The explanatory models held by both patients and providers should be elucidated and commonly held values shared as the basis for identifying strategies for decision-making. A simple strategy to determine the explanatory model of patients is to inquire into their beliefs about the etiology and meanings (including fears) of illnesses or symptoms and into what goals or outcomes they hope for from any available treatments (37). Next, patients and families should be asked to share the values or moral principles that they feel need to be upheld when they make important decisions. Lastly, physicians should clearly understand the principles, both personal and professional, that guide their ethical positions.

The principles upheld by Mr. Choi's physician represented ethical and legal standards of medical practice. These principles reflect Western philosophical and legal traditions. Moreover, physicians in similar situations may feel pressure, both moral and legal, to promote these standards. The Choi family, on the other hand, placed a high value on family honor and the fulfillment of duties. The strategy for resolution in this case involved a reframing of the notion of autonomy (10,37). The patient was offered the right to choose whether to be treated autonomously, an option that allowed the physician a way to honor both her own and the Choi family's values.

Attitudinal Aspects of Culturally Effective Care

CASE 3-3. AN AFRICAN-AMERICAN MAN WITH ADVANCED PROSTATE CANCER, AND THE IMPACT OF MISTRUST ON DISCUSSIONS OF MEDICAL FUTILITY

Communication concerning end-of-life issues had always been difficult between Lawrence Byrd, an African American, and his primary care physician, a European-American who was 20 years his junior. The physician had cared for Mr. Byrd since his initial diagnosis of cancer and had found him to be an angry and rather mistrustful patient. The provider had made many attempts to improve his relationship with Mr. Byrd, including suggesting that they be on a first-name basis in an effort to enhance familiarity. However, Mr. Byrd refused to call the doctor by his first name, although the physician persisted in referring to the patient as "Lawrence."

The physician assumed that the patient's insistence on aggressive care might have stemmed from a failure to understand the limits of medical technology. Consequently, the physician used every clinical encounter as an opportunity to discuss the value of limiting treatment, emphasizing the desirability of palliative care in light of his view of medical futility. These discussions, perceived as patronizing by Mr. Byrd, were often unproductive, leaving both the patient and provider frustrated.

In order to improve the doctor-patient relationship, the physician asked a member of his medical group, an African-American physician, for her insights into the case. After reviewing the medical history and hearing the physician's impressions of "Lawrence," the colleague suggested that he consider ways in which his behaviors had seemed patronizing and disrespectful to the patient. She noted that calling an African-American elder by his first name is considered highly impertinent. This, coupled with continual discussions of medical futility could have been interpreted as a devaluation of Mr. Byrd's life. Lastly, she suggested that the patient's insistence on aggressive therapy could be related to African-American values about the sanctity of life, not a lack of education.

At his next visit, the physician, addressing the patient as "Mr. Byrd," stated his concerns about possible past misunderstandings. He then respectfully inquired whether he indeed had experienced racism or a devaluing of his life in the health care system. Mr. Byrd shared stories of incidents in the hospital and emergency settings in which his requests for pain medication went unanswered. He also revealed injustices he had experienced during his life, including situations in the clinic in which he felt ill-treated and not valued. Mr. Byrd additionally told the physician that the suggestions to not consider curative treatment because of medical futility seemed to him to be a discussion about cost, which further confirmed his belief that his life was devalued. He explained that his signing of an advance directive requesting full support was an effort to protect his survival.

Unaware of these incidents of abuse, the physician apologized for any insensitivity that he may have perpetrated and shared with Mr. Byrd that he did value him as a patient. He stated that Mr. Byrd's well being was important and that he would continue to hold this value as they proceeded in exploring all the possibilities for his care. He informed the patient that when they reached a point where the fight for his life would tilt the balance toward more suffering, he would not abandon him. Rather, he promised he would do all that he could to make sure that Mr. Byrd would not experience unnecessary pain.

Identified Problems

The physician's intentions to help Mr. Byrd were genuine but initially ineffective and were met, in turn, with hostility and mistrust. By insisting that they be on a first-name basis—a value understood and held within his own cultural framework—the doctor failed to address the values of respect for elders held by African Americans. The physician's assumption that the insistence on aggressive care was due to a lack of education might suggest implicit negative associations about race that may exist outside of the awareness of those who are otherwise against discrimination (38). Add to this that in both clinical encounters and in epidemiologic research, concepts such as race, ethnicity, culture, gender, age, and other interactive features are often poorly understood and erroneously conflated with notions of class, socioeconomics, and education (36,39,40). Such confusions can contribute to negative ethnic or racial stereotypes. By assuming poor health literacy as an explanation and failing to ascertain other reasons behind Mr. Byrd's desire for aggressive care, the physician may have compounded the patient's suspicions of racism (41).

Strategies for Effective Care

A physician's intentions to do good may not necessarily provide insight into the lived experience of the patient. In the case of Mr. Byrd, cultural sensitivity was needed to recognize potential obstacles to effective palliative care. By consulting a cultural "insider," one who understood both the medical and cultural issues involved in this case, the physician was able to identify behaviors that were barriers to effective care.

It is important for physicians not to construe situations of mistrust as a problem inherent to an individual or groups. Doing so fails to address situations of untrustworthiness often experienced by minorities. For example, Mr. Byrd shared incidents where his requests for pain medication were left unattended. Inadequately addressing pain control based on patient ethnicity is a reality for some African-American patients. Studies demonstrating this outcome further highlight the untrustworthiness of medical systems to meet the needs of minorities (24-26). Recognition of mistrust should alert providers to inquire into actual incidents of discrimination or abuse. Patients can be asked, "Have you ever experienced a time when your requests for pain medication were not adequately addressed?" or "Have you or has anyone you know been treated with insensitivity or disrespect while seeking medical care?" Inquiring in a respectful manner, followed by a willingness to believe that the patient's experience is real for them, can be the first steps in establishing and/or restoring patient trust. When incidents that can engender mistrust are reported, follow-up through appropriate channels may be necessary to prevent future events.

The cases presented here highlight the need for culturally effective care that includes both technical competence and attitudinal sensitivity to negotiate the complexities of difference. Although working with cultural differences at the end of life may require providers to expand the possibilities of what constitutes a "good death," many of the practical skills needed in a cross-cultural context do not differ from those needed to serve any patient or family who is facing death (36,42). These clinical tasks are not easy in any context, but through enhancing communication skills, offering sensitivity and competence in both treatment and palliative care, and respecting differences in values that support end-of-life decisions, patients of all communities and their families can be well cared for through the dying process.

Summary

What motivates and influences us in life is significant and instrumental at the end of life as well. For some persons, the end of life may provide an opportunity for deep reflection on the meaning of life and of the value of family and loved ones. For others, the process of dying can be an alienating and frightening experience. Community, religious, and cultural ties, including spiritual beliefs and practices, may provide a source of great comfort as patients and families prepare for death. It is important for providers to inquire into cultural preferences or taboos that may affect care at the end of life. They should become aware of the specific beliefs and practices of the populations they serve, always remembering to inquire whether their particular patients value these beliefs. As the three cases have sought to illustrate, knowing the larger context of an individual's life can greatly aid in understanding critical issues at play during the dying process.

Failure to incorporate differences in beliefs, values, and preferences in communication, clinical care practices, and ethical decision-making will hinder opportunities for effective end-of-life care. Providers should cultivate attitudes and behaviors that recognize and respect cultural diversity. This includes recognizing the dual nature of their own cultural agency—that which is embedded within the culture of medicine and that which acts as mediator between the worlds of doctor and patient. By incorporating cultural sensitivity and competency into palliative care practices, physicians can provide better care for all patients at the end of life.

Acknowledgements

We gratefully acknowledge the generous support for our work in cultural diversity and end-of-life care from the American Foundation for AIDS Research (1772), National Institutes of Health (R01 NR029060), Open Society Institute Project on Death in America, the Robert Wood Johnson Foundation, State of California AIDS Research Project (R95-ST-188), the Greenwall Foundation, and the University of California, San Francisco, AIDS Clinical Research Center.

REFERENCES

1. **Field MJ, Cassel CK, Eds.** Approaching Death: Improving Care at the End of Life. Washington, DC: National Academy Press; 1997.
2. **Orr RD, Marshall PA, Osborn J.** Cross-cultural considerations in clinical ethics consultations. Arch Fam Med. 1995;4:159-64.
3. **Carrillo JE, Green AR, Betancourt JR.** Cross-cultural primary care: a patient-based approach. Ann Intern Med. 1999;130:829-34.
4. **Culhane-Pera KA, Reif C, Egli E, et al.** A curriculum for multicultural education in family medicine. Fam Med. 1997;29:719-23.
5. **Lavizzo-Mourey R, Mackenzie ER.** Cultural competence: essential measurements of quality for managed care organizations. Ann Intern Med. 1996;124:919-21.
6. **Tervalon M, Murray-Garcia J.** Cultural humility versus cultural competence: a critical distinction in defining physician training outcomes in multicultural education. J Health Care Poor Underserved. 1998;9:117-25.
7. **Zweifler J, Gonzalez AM.** Teaching residents to care for culturally diverse populations. Acad Med. 1998;73:1056-61.

8. **Committee on Pediatric Workforce.** Culturally effective pediatric care: education and training issues. Pediatrics. 1999;103:167-70.
9. **Blackhall LJ, Murphy ST, Frank G, et al.** Ethnicity and attitudes toward patient autonomy. JAMA. 1995;274:820-5.
10. **Hern HE, Koenig BA, Moore LJ, Marshall PA.** The difference that culture can make in end-of-life decision-making. Camb Q Healthc Ethics. 1998;7:27-40.
11. **Murphy ST, Palmer JM, Azen S, et al.** Ethnicity and advance directives. J Law Med Ethics. 1996;24:108-17.
12. **Marshall PA, Koenig BA, Barnes DM, Davis AJ.** Multiculturalism, bioethics, and end-of-life care: case narratives of Latino cancer patients. In: Monagle J, Thomasma D, Eds. Health Care Ethics: Critical Issues for the 21st Century. Gaithersburg, MD: Aspen Publishers; 1998;421-31.
13. **Fox RC.** The sociology of bioethics. In: The Sociology of Medicine: A Participant Observer's View. Englewood Cliffs, NJ: Prentice-Hall; 1989; 224-76.
14. **Fox RC.** The evolution of American bioethics: a social perspective. In: Weisz G, Ed. Social Science Perspectives on Medical Ethics. London: Kluwer Academic Publishers; 1990;201-17.
15. **Geissler EM.** Pocket Guide to Cultural Assessment. St. Louis: Mosby; 1998.
16. **Lipson JG, Dibble, SL, Minarik PA, Eds.** Culture and Nursing Care: A Pocket Guide. San Francisco: UCSF Nursing Press; 1996.
17. **Lock M.** Education and self reflection: teaching about culture, health and illness. In: Masi R, et al, Eds. Health and Cultures: Exploring the Relationships. Oakville, Ontario, Canada: Mosaic Press; 1993;139.
18. **Doyle D, Hanks GWC, MacDonald N.** Oxford Textbook of Palliative Medicine, 2nd ed. New York: Oxford University Press; 1998.
19. **Storey P.** Primer of Palliative Care, 2nd ed. Gainesville, FL: American Academy of Hospice and Palliative Medicine; 1996.
20. **MacDonald N.** Palliative Medicine: A Case-Based Manual. New York: Oxford University Press; 1998.
21. **Poulson J.** Impact of cultural difference in care of the terminally ill. In: MacDonald N, Ed. Palliative Medicine: A Case-Based Manual. New York: Oxford University Press; 1998;244-52.
22. **Bates MS, Sanchez-Ayendez M.** The effects of the cultural context of health care on treatment of and response to chronic pain and illness. Soc Sci Med. 1997;45:1433-7.
23. **Irish DP, Lundquist KF, Nelsen VJ.** Ethnic Variations in Dying, Death, and Grief: Diversity in Universality. Washington, DC: Taylor and Francis; 1993.
24. **Todd KH, Samaroo N, Hoffman JR.** Ethnicity as a risk factor for inadequate emergency department analgesia. JAMA. 1993;269:1537-9.
25. **Cleeland CS, Gonin R, Baez L, et al.** Pain and treatment of pain in minority patients with cancer. The Eastern Cooperative Oncology Group Minority Outpatient Pain Study. Ann Intern Med. 1997;127:813-6.
26. **Engle VF, Fox-Hill E, Graney MJ.** The experience of living-dying in a nursing home: self-reports of black and white older adults. J Am Geriatr Soc. 1998;46:1091-6.

27. **Eisenbruch M.** Cross-cultural aspects of bereavement. I: A conceptual framework for comparative analysis. Cult Med Psychiatry. 1984;8:283-309.
28. **Eisenbruch M.** Cross-cultural aspects of bereavement. II: Ethnic and cultural variations in the development of bereavement practices. Cult Med Psychiatry. 1984;8:315-47.
29. **Perkins HS.** Cultural differences and ethical issues in the problem of autopsy requests. Texas Med. 1991;87:72-7.
30. **Marshall PA, Koenig BA, Grifhorst P, van Ewijk M.** Ethical issues in immigrant health care and clinical research. In: Loue S, Ed. Handbook of Immigrant Health. New York: Plenum Press; 1998:203-6.
31. **Welsh M, Feldman MD.** Cross-cultural communication. In: Feldman MD, Christensen JF, Eds. Behavioral Medicine in Primary Care: A Practical Guide. Stamford, CT: Appleton and Lange; 1997:97-108.
32. **Gavagan T, Martinez A.** Presentation of recent torture survivors to a family practice center. J Fam Prac. 1997;44:209-12.
33. **Gamble VN.** A legacy of distrust: African Americans and medical research. Am J Prevent Med. 1993;1993:35-8.
34. **Haffner L.** Translation is not enough: interpreting in a medical setting. West J Med. 1992;157:255-9.
35. **Triandis HC, Marin G, Lisansky J, et al.** Simpatia as a cultural script of Hispanics. J Pers Soc Psychol. 1984;47:1363-75.
36. **Koenig BA, Gates-Williams J.** Understanding cultural difference in caring for dying patients. West J Med. 1995;163:244-9.
37. **Kleinman A, Eisenberg L, Good B.** Culture, illness, and care: clinical lessons from anthropologic and cross-cultural research. Ann Intern Med. 1978; 88:251-8.
38. **Dovidio JF, Kawakami K, Johnson C, et al.** On the nature of prejudice: automatic and controlled processes. J Exp Psychol. 1997; 33:510-40.
39. **Bhopal R.** Is research into ethnicity and health racist, unsound, or important science? BMJ. 1997;314:1751-6.
40. **Bhopal R.** Spectre of racism in health and health care: lessons from history and the United States. BMJ. 1998;316:1970-3.
41. **Dula A.** African American suspicion of the health care system is justified: what do we do about it? Camb Q Healthc Ethics. 1994;3:347-57.
42. **Block SD, Bernier GM, Crawley LM, et al.** Incorporating palliative care into primary care education. National Consensus Conference on Medical Education for Care Near the End of Life. J Gen Intern Med. 1998;13:768-73.

CHAPTER 4

Beyond Symptom Management: Physician Roles and Responsibility in Palliative Care

IRA R. BYOCK, MD • ARTHUR CAPLAN, PhD •
LOIS SNYDER, JD

Role of the Physician in Caring Beyond Cure

Chronic illnesses are now the most common causes of death in the United States (1). For many patients, medical care can slow the course of the illness and improve quality of life, but as illness advances, continued life-prolonging interventions can impose increasing burdens and offer diminishing returns. Often, there is no clear point of transition. The lack of reliable physiological markers for determining when a patient is "dying" remains an obstacle to research and policy development to improve end-of-life care (2-6).

Despite the inherent uncertainty of identifying when precisely patients are approaching life's end, physicians must provide care that meets recognized clinical standards and responds to the needs of patients (7). Caring for people approaching death will always draw on the art and humanity of the practitioner. The responsibility of ensuring excellent medical care for the dying patient lies with the attending physician.

Recent studies have documented serious deficiencies in access to and quality of care in the months, weeks, and days before death (1,8-10). Correcting deficiencies and raising practice standards and expectations within the professional culture and developing improved models for end-of-life care delivery are important challenges.

Principles and Practice of Palliative Care

In practice, the transition from life-prolonging to palliative treatment is often gradual and may only be recognized in retrospect. The anonymous 16th-century aphorism, "To Cure Sometimes, To Relieve Often, To Comfort Always" (11), describes an integrated continuum of care that sets a standard for physicians and the health care system to meet. In providing treatment to enhance comfort and support to improve the quality of patients' lives, physicians who care for patients with progressive illness routinely incorporate a palliative approach to care within their range of practice.

In current usage, "palliative care" also refers to an area of distinct practice delivered by clinicians with particular expertise and by specialized teams, such as hospice programs or hospital-based palliative care services (11). In the United Kingdom, palliative medicine has formal status as a medical specialty. In the United States, the Institute of Medicine recommended, "Palliative care should become, if not a medical specialty, at least a defined area of expertise, education, and research" (1). Whether the term is used to connote a general approach or to refer to an area of specialized practice, palliative care does not represent a departure from the tenets of general medicine. It is, instead, distinguished by its strong emphasis on specific principles, such as alleviation of suffering, symptom management, good communication, and supportive counseling related to illness, disability, and limited prognosis.

Specialized programs of palliative care rely on an interdisciplinary team model composed of professionals and trained volunteers (12). Each member of the team contributes particular skills and areas of emphasis (13). Within this interdisciplinary team dynamic, the physician's area of concentration includes symptom management, as well as continued, appropriate application of disease-modifying therapy. The patient with his or her family is the focus of care, with "family" being operationally defined as the people who are most important to the patient, and to whom the patient is most important. Dying is regarded as an inherently difficult, but normal, stage in the life of individuals and families. In contrast to problem-based medicine, a patient need not have acute or active "problems" to warrant evaluation and intervention. A diagnosis of progressive, incurable illness or any constellation of medical problems that result in progressive disability or an eventually terminal prognosis are indications for palliative care. By identifying quality of life as a central focus, attention is shifted to patients' subjective experience. During the initial period of bereavement, typically through the first anniversary of the person's death, palliative care offers support for the family and screens for instances of complicated grief requiring referral for formal counseling (Table 4-1) (14-16).

Specialized palliative care services and programs expand the resource base and complete a full spectrum of essential health care services (17). In the United States, hospice is the best-known delivery model for palliative care. The most experienced and skillful hospice programs provide a "best practice" standard against which to assess the quality of palliative and end-of-life care (18).

Relief of physical distress is the first priority for palliative care. Symptom management requires an organized, ongoing approach that is careful, comprehensive, and, when necessary, intensive. Pain is a cardinal symptom associated with late-stages of cancer, advanced HIV infection, and progressive, crippling diseases. However, dyspnea, nausea, profound weakness, and delirium are all common sources of physical distress among dying patients (19-21). Specialists in medical and radiation oncology, anesthesiology, neurology, surgery, and neurosurgery commonly contribute to the team process of palliative care. The "intensive" nature of symptom-alleviating (interventions such as neurolytic blocks for unrelenting neuropathic pain or sedation for management of otherwise uncontrolled terminal agitation) is properly limited only by patient-imposed restrictions.

Suffering for the dying patient often extends beyond physical distress, involving emotional, social, and spiritual dimensions. As function wanes and the activities, roles, and responsibilities that have given meaning to life fall away, a sense of impending disintegration and loss

---

Table 4-1. Precepts of Palliative Care.

- Ethical decision-making that respects patient autonomy and the role of family or legal surrogates
- Interdisciplinary team approach to care
- Patient with his or her family as the unit of care
- Effective and (when necessary) intensive symptom management
- Dying understood as a time of life; improving quality of life as a primary goal
- Recognition of the importance of the "inner life" of the patient
- Bereavement support to family during initial period of grieving

of meaning may be experienced (22,23). Clinicians caring for patients who are struggling with issues of life closure best serve the dying person and family by staying involved, listening, and expressing a willingness to support the person in exploring his or her own answers (24). Sources of emotional and spiritual distress can be acknowledged, assessed, and effectively responded to without requiring the assignment of psychological diagnoses. Beyond alleviation of physical symptoms and psychoemotional distress, physicians can help patients to live as fully as possible and complete tasks they identify as most important during this poignant time.

CASE 4-1. A 67-YEAR-OLD ATTORNEY WITH NON-SMALL CELL LUNG CARCINOMA, METASTATIC TO THE BRAIN

Mr. Baker is a 67-year-old attorney. Ten months ago he noticed a subtle change in right-sided fine motor control while writing. When his secretary questioned his signature on a letter, he made an appointment with Dr. Jones, his internist. During that week he also became aware of intermittent difficulty with word searching. Dr. Jones noted slight right-sided weakness. A magnetic resonance imaging scan revealed a 2.5-cm left parietal-temporal lesion and a smaller left posterior lobe lesion. Chest x-ray showed a solitary left upper lobe nodule. A transbronchial needle biopsy confirmed the diagnosis of non-small cell lung carcinoma, metastatic to the brain.

Whole-brain radiation was promptly begun and tolerated without problems. Mr. Baker's neurologic symptoms rapidly resolved. A consulting medical oncologist presented the risks and potential benefits of combination chemotherapy for his condition (25,26). Mr. Baker decided against chemotherapy.

Mr. Baker has continued to see Dr. Jones for monthly checkups. He has not had further focal neurologic symptoms or acute problems; however, gradual weight loss, diminished energy, and exercise tolerance have slowly worsened.

Four days ago, Mr. Baker developed significantly increased low back pain and 2 days ago noted bilateral weakness in his legs. Contacted by phone, Dr. Jones sent Mr. Baker to the emergency room of the University hospital, where he was evaluated by Dr. Young and a first-year resident.

After discussion with Dr. Jones, morphine was given for immediate comfort and Mr. Baker was admitted. Dr. Young elicited a report of recent onset of urinary incontinence and "numbness" in his feet, and examination uncovered 3-over-5 lower extremity weakness, abnormal plantar responses, and diminished rectal sphincter tone. An emergency magnetic resonance imaging scan revealed impending lumbar spinal cord compression caused by a metastatic lesion and an additional midthoracic vertebral metastasis. A bone scan detailed another probable lesion in his right proximal femur. High-dose intravenous dexamethasone was administered. Urgent neurosurgery and radiation oncology consultations were obtained and, after discussions with Dr. Jones and Mr. Baker, local radiotherapy to the vertebral metastases and the femoral lesion was begun on an emergency basis (27). Mr. Baker's pain rapidly improves and neurologic symptoms stabilize, but lower extremity weakness persists.

Mr. Baker wants all available information and to make his own decisions. Each day Dr. Jones and Dr. Young review the latest test results with him. Dr. Jones answers all his patient's questions in nontechnical terms. He suggests that it is now time to consider involving the hospice team in his care. Mr. Baker initially bristles, "Are you giving up on me, Doctor?", then bluntly asks how much longer he has to live. Dr. Jones assures Mr. Baker that he is not going to stop caring for him and responds that, though it is always difficult to estimate with certainty, his life expectancy is probably weeks to at most a few months. During the conversation, Mr. Baker reluctantly agrees to a hospice referral.

During the intake interview with the hospice nurse case manager and social worker, Mr. Baker's living situation and social history are reviewed. His law practice has always consumed most of his time. He has been divorced twice and lives alone. He and his first wife, Margaret, maintain contact. Their three children live out of state. A son and elder daughter are each married with young children, and a younger daughter attends graduate school. Mr. Baker's strongest wish is to stay at home until he dies.

Mr. Baker is transferred to a rehabilitation unit while receiving daily radiation therapy. Oral long-acting morphine controls his back pain. Baclofen is started for leg spasms and lorazepam is available for intermittent anxiety. Occasional nausea is treated with perchlorperazine (28). Dexamethasone is tapered and prednisone 20 mg per day is begun as an adjunct for analgesia and to improve appetite and general well-being (29). Physical and occupational therapy are begun, including transfer skills and the use of assistive devices, so that Mr. Baker can continue to dress and toilet himself.

Mr. Baker complains little. His most serious symptomatic distress occurs when, because of an oversight, no bowel regimen is prescribed and constipation is overlooked for 5 days, resulting in painful abdominal cramps. Multiple enemas and digital disimpaction resolve the problem. Mr. Baker tells Dr. Jones that the experience is an assault on his dignity. Thereafter stool softeners with stimulant laxatives are prescribed for routine use and doses of oral sorbitol adjusted on a daily basis (11).

Mr. Baker's children arrive from out of town. Before discharge, a family meeting is held. Margaret agrees to participate in his care. Hospice volunteers are assigned to help with household chores, errands, and transportation.

Dr. Jones asks the hospice nurse to administer a quality-of-life survey designed to assess the subjective experience of patients with far-advanced illness (30). Mr. Baker's responses suggest feelings of guilt and low self-worth. These issues are explored by the hospice social worker and in sessions with the hospice chaplain in which, to his family's surprise, Mr. Baker shows great interest.

During a second family meeting, Mr. Baker and his children talk openly about their disappointments and fears. Mr. Baker asserts that, despite his law career, in his heart his children have always been most important to him.

In the weeks that follow, the family spends considerable time visiting. Generalized weakness progresses and Mr. Baker becomes bed-bound. At the chaplain's suggestion, Mr. Baker, with help, tapes several hours of stories from his childhood as a gift to his grandchildren.

On one visit in which Dr. Young is present, Dr. Jones asks Mr. Baker if he feels there would be anything left undone if he were to die suddenly. After a moment of thought, he smiles wryly and responds, "Oh, I'd like to live 20 more years, but the truth is that everything is in place."

Two months after coming home, Mr. Baker abruptly becomes confused and unable to speak or swallow. Emergency evaluation by the hospice nurse confirms increased right-sided weakness. In phone consultation with Dr. Jones, the symptoms are attributed to a probable intracranial hemorrhage or other cerebral-vascular compromise. Consistent with Mr. Baker's wishes and the plan of care, no diagnostic workup is initiated. Oral medications are discontinued. A low-dose subcutaneous morphine infusion is administered, to replace oral narcotics, providing for continued analgesia and preventing possible withdrawal symptoms. Additional rescue bolus doses are prescribed pro re nata for signs of discomfort such as grimacing or muscle stiffening on turning. A small dose of subcutaneous midazolam is administered by continuous infusion as an antispasmotic, an anxiolytic, and a prophylaxis for possible seizures (31,32). Dr. Jones is unable to visit but calls Margaret, inquiring about Mr. Baker's status and level of comfort, and reviews the current plan of care and orders with the on-call hospice nurse.

The family gathers at the home. Mr. Baker is mostly somnolent, although he intermittently becomes alert, acknowledging his family. He is often touched, his hand held and his skin cleansed or oiled, while family members talk. They each say goodbye. Mr. Baker dies quietly the next morning with his family present.

Dr. Jones is out of town the day of the memorial service but sends a condolence card. He encourages Dr. Young to attend. During a eulogy given by Mr. Baker's son, Dr. Young is moved to be acknowledged by name.

Dr. Young confides to Dr. Jones that this case has been one of the most profound clinical experiences he has had. Later that spring, Dr. Young arranges to spend a full day attending the hospice interdisciplinary team meeting and making rounds with Dr. Jones. He is surprised by the range of diagnoses among the hospice patients, including several with advanced emphysema and congestive heart failure, two with far-advanced dementia, and a patient with renal failure who had just stopped dialysis. Dr. Young remarks about the appreciation expressed by patients and families for the importance of this time in their lives. He decides to take a month-long elective hospice rotation in his third year.

Six months after Mr. Baker's death, the hospice team continues to make intermittent contact with Margaret and his children. Margaret has joined a bereavement support group.

Discussion

Mr. Baker was fortunate to have a physician who knew him well, was adept at palliative interventions, and who recognized an important role in supporting patients at the end of life. Medical house staff frequently encounter patients who have lacked consistent medical care before an acute hospitalization. Within the context of bedside and specialty rounds, attending physicians typically focus on the disease-modifying treatment and, to an increasing extent, on symptom management. Living situations of patients and families may only be assessed to the extent they impact discharge planning and patient placement. Within teaching hospitals, medical direction for incurably ill patients' care may be delegated to interns and resident physicians. Patients discharged to nursing homes commonly have primary care transferred to physicians covering the receiving institution.

In current practice, the subjective experience of dying patients or their families may only become a priority for treating physicians when suffering gives rise to disruptive or otherwise demanding behavior. Over-reliance on a problem-based approach can lead to an unfortunate constriction in the scope of physician practice. To confine medicine's focus to physiological interventions is to limit the art, and heart, of medicine. A physician who avoids imposing a "hospice philosophy" on patients in order to maintain a value-neutral therapeutic stance is mistaken. Although palliative care is value-laden, it is no more so than prevailing modes of disease-modifying treatment. Limiting patient choices constrains their ability, and their right, to make autonomous decisions.

As Case 4-1 illustrates, life-prolonging and palliative care need not be an "either/or" choice. At the time of diagnosis, no curative treatment was available for Mr. Baker. Care continued and, when symptoms developed, prompt diagnostic workups were conducted, consultants were involved, and appropriate disease-modifying and symptomatic interventions promptly begun. Life-prolonging and comfort measures were provided concomitantly, reflecting the concordant nature of these goals. Mr. Baker's authority to make final treatment decisions was respected.

Dr. Jones' plan of care extended beyond ensuring that his patient was fully informed and providing meticulous symptom management. He directed an organized assessment of the impact of physical discomfort, functional limitations, and awareness of death's approach on Mr. Baker's emotional well-being and his subjective quality of life. He provided anticipatory guidance and mobilized resources to support his patient in adapting to this difficult life transition. And he extended this support to Mr. Baker's family in their caregiving and adjustment to their impending loss.

Dr. Jones helped Mr. Baker identify "things left undone" and identify meaningful and realistic goals. He listened. He related stories of previous patients and families who had used similar times to express mutual forgiveness, reinforce their appreciation and affection for one another, and undertake similar opportunities for closure.

When Mr. Baker was admitted to hospice care, the hospice nurse assumed the role of case manager. Dr. Jones retained leadership of his patient's health care team and final authority for his care.

Dr. Jones was conscious of the learning opportunity that Mr. Baker's care afforded Dr. Young. In his role as clinical instructor, he provided Dr. Young with information and the reasoning behind appropriate symptom-alleviating medications and interventions. He modeled skills in communication, including listening. In treatment and in counseling, Dr. Jones conveyed to Dr. Young the importance of caring for patients as they die. These are important aspects of the role of clinical instructors and warrant consideration in processes of advancement for academic physicians.

Barriers to Palliative Care

Not all patients are as receptive to this type of care and support as Mr. Baker and his family, and not all cases are as well managed. Barriers to providing good palliative care exist (Table 4-2). Perhaps the most obvious barrier encountered by busy physicians is too little time to do all that they would like to do for patients and families. Excellent palliative care requires more than knowledge of symptom alleviation and basic counseling skills; it requires time to impart information and time to listen. Meaningful communication regarding matters of dying and options for care requires time to explore whatever questions patients and family members may have.

Our societal tendency to avoid the subjects of dying and death is another barrier to communicating with and counseling people who are suffering emotional, psychosocial, or spiritual distress related to advanced illness. The life-saving orientation of mainstream medicine also tends to reinforce a denial of death (1). Physicians may be reluctant to refer to palliative care and hospice programs, fearing that patients will interpret the suggestion as abandonment, as Mr. Baker initially did, and patients and families may be reluctant to accept a referral, viewing it as a loss of hope.

Current regulatory and payment structures, epitomized by eligibility criteria under the Medicare hospice benefit, reflect and reinforce a false dichotomy between life-prolonging and palliative care. System-based limitations of this nature impose an unnecessary, "either/or" choice on patients and families and challenge clinicians to combine measures to extend life and interventions to improve the quality of life in a manner that is seamless and at all points consistent with the cultural values and personal goals of the people they serve.

Table 4-2. Barriers to Palliative Care.

Time limitations
Barriers within the culture of medicine
  Life-prolonging and curative orientation of medicine
  Death as a "bad outcome"
Clinical barriers
  Prognostic uncertainty
  Insufficient knowledge and skills
  Inadequate prescribing for pain control
Inadequate physician-patient communication
Ethnic, cultural, and religious challenges
Legal, regulatory, procedural, and financial barriers
Education and training deficiencies

Rather than conflicting, the cultural differences between life-prolonging and palliative care can effectively complement one another. For many patients and families, relentless disease progression and increasing disability gradually erode denial of the approach of life's end. As with Mr. Baker's appreciation of the hospice chaplain's visits, interest in and openness to addressing issues of meaning or spiritual connection often surprises those who knew the patient well before illness. When life-prolongation is exclusively pursued, a discrepancy can arise between clinician goals and plans of care and patient-centered priorities. Physicians who, for instance, assume that mundane details of bathing and transportation or psychosocial tasks are not their concerns, may neglect the needs that patients may feel are most important. Physicians may miss opportunities to suggest involvement of consultants and valuable resources such as home health aides, social workers, and clergy and leave patients and families feeling unsupported in the very issues that most affect their quality of life.

Problems related to health care systems, logistics, and even financing often can be alleviated by individualized, case-by-base advocacy and coordination. These services are, themselves, time-intensive. Although physicians can assist in these efforts, care management is often overseen by a primary nurse or social worker. Clerical staff also may help patients gain access to needed services and coordinate visits, transportation, and home-based care.

Working in their own health systems and communities, physicians can view these barriers as opportunities for institutional and programmatic quality-improvement efforts. Collectively, the medical profession can provide leadership by reducing barriers to excellent, inclusive care for dying patients and their families through professional education, research, clinical quality improvement, policy development, and participation in public education and advocacy.

Preservation of Opportunity: A Clinical Role and Responsibility

Although symptom management and relief of suffering are the first priorities for palliative care, they are not the ultimate goals. The experience of living with a progressive illness affects every dimension of a person's life: physical, social, emotional, and spiritual. Consistent with ethical tenets of medicine, patient and family priorities properly guide treatment priorities reflected in the plan of care. To avoid interfering with an important, a poignant, and a potentially meaningful time in the lives of dying patients and families, whenever possible, expediency in the scheduling of medical tests and delivery of treatments should be subordinated to the personal goals of those being served. Medication schedules can be adjusted, home-based services initiated, and care coordinated among local providers. In hospital and intensive care unit settings, deliberate attention is warranted to minimize blood draws and x-rays and related intrusions and distractions. Routine measures, such as daily weights, measurement of intake and output, cardiac and oxygen saturation monitoring, and blood pressure readings, which no longer contribute to an individual patient's current clinical priorities and goals, may be discontinued. Meals need not be delivered to patients who are not eating. A sign on the door, alerting visitors to check with the patient's nurse before entering, can help preserve a semblance of intimacy for a hospitalized patient and family.

Unlike sudden death, dying of a progressive illness offers the chance to "get one's affairs in order." Financial and legal affairs can be settled. People have a chance to say things that would have been left unsaid if death had come abruptly. They have the opportunity to heal strained relationships. There is a chance to get one's most important interpersonal affairs in order, saying: "Forgive me, I forgive you, Thank you, I love you, Goodbye" (33,34). Relationships can become complete, even if they are not imminently ending.

Dying from a progressive illness presents opportunities for reminiscence and life-review that can facilitate life completion (35-38). Providers can help patients and families use activities to deepen the sense of meaning about the life lived. Story telling can be more than a pleasant pastime, becoming a means to transmit one's special knowledge and wisdom to others (39). Families of patients with advanced, incurable illness can benefit from the chance to express their love in words and through the care they provide. For the patient who desires spiritual exploration, palliative care providers can acknowledge and encourage the process. Patients are well served by clinicians who are willing and able to remain emotionally involved, visiting as time permits, if only to listen in a non-judgmental manner.

Barriers to Life Closure

Although a number of valuable opportunities exist during the time of living identified as "dying," they are just that—opportunities. Developmental assessments must not, however, become criteria on which a patient or family's worth is judged. Some issues of personal and family history will not lend themselves to forgiveness, and extremely difficult clinical or social situations may afford no chance for introspection or the intimate communication required for reconciliation. Sudden death, critical care settings, severe, uncontrolled symptoms, serious family dysfunction, social circumstances, poverty, or psychosocial problems all represent significant challenges to a satisfying sense of life closure (Table 4-3).

Table 4-3. Barriers to Satisfactory Life Closure.

Severe, uncontrolled symptoms
  Pain
  Dyspnea
  Nausea
  Confusion
Poverty
  Housing
  Transportation
  Medical care
Family and social support
  Family dysfunction
  Child abuse
  Physical and sexual violence
  Active drug and alcohol abuse
  Mental illness
Critical care environments
  Constant activity and noise
  Traditional emphasis on technology
  Prolongation of life; relative inattention to suffering
  Surrounded by others in active fight for life
Sudden death
  Lack of preparation; anticipation
  Often lack of ongoing medical relationships
  More complicated bereavement

Clinicians are challenged to avoid the nihilism that can undermine valuable opportunities for dying patients and families while averting guilt or recriminations within families when, for whatever reasons, such opportunities remain unfulfilled. Difficult situations and the myriad sources of suffering that people encounter highlight the importance of the collective efforts, and potential synergistic efficacy, of clinical teams (12). The more complex and troublesome a case becomes, the more pressing becomes the need for involving the resources of the palliative care team.

Summary

When cure is no longer possible and life prolongation is a fleeting goal, the ongoing process of care presents an important and potentially satisfying role for physicians. Working with a team of prepared, committed providers, physicians can practice and model care that integrates life-prolongation with comfort and patient-defined goals. In this manner, patients can be helped to live fully and die well.

REFERENCES

1. **Institute of Medicine.** Approaching Death. Washington, DC: National Academy Press; 1997.
2. **Brody H, Lynn J.** The physician's responsibility under the new Medicare reimbursement for hospice care. N Engl J Med. 1984;310:920.
3. **Lynn J, Harrell FE, et al.** Prognoses of seriously ill hospitalized patients on the days before death: implications for patient care and public policy. New Horiz. 1997;5:56-61.
4. **Lynn J, Teno JM, Harrell FE.** Accurate prognostications of death: opportunities and challenges for clinicians. West J Med. 1995;163:250.
5. **Knaus WA, Harrell FE, Lynn J, et al.** The SUPPORT prognostic model: objective estimates of survival for seriously ill hospitalized patients. Ann Intern Med. 1995;122:191.
6. **Lynn J, Harrell FE, Cohn F, et al.** Defining the "terminally ill": Insights from SUPPORT. Duquesne Law Review. 1996;35:311-36.
7. **American College of Physicians.** Ethics manual. 4th ed. Ann Intern Med. 1998;128:576-94.
8. **Knaus WA, Lynn J, Teno J, et al.** A controlled trial to improve care for seriously ill hospitalized patients. JAMA. 1995;274:1591-8.
9. **Cleeland CS, Gonin R, Hatfield AK, et al.** Pain and its treatment in outpatients with metastatic cancer. N Engl J Med. 1994;330:592-6.

10. **Bernabei R, Gambassi G, Lapane K, et al.** Management of pain in elderly patients with cancer. JAMA. 1998;279:1877-82.
11. **Doyle D, Hanks GWC, MacDonald H, Eds.** Oxford Textbook of Palliative Medicine. 2nd ed. New York: Oxford University Press; 1997.
12. **Cummings I.** The interdisciplinary team. In: Doyle D, Hanks GWC, MacDonald H, Eds. Oxford Textbook of Palliative Medicine. 2nd ed. New York: Oxford University Press; 1997.
13. **Lattanzi-Licht M, Mahoney JJ, Miller GW.** The Hospice Choice. New York: Simon and Schuster; 1998.
14. **Canadian Palliative Care Association.** Palliative Care: Towards Standardized Principles of Practice. 1995.
15. **Last Acts Task Force, Robert Wood Johnson Foundation.** Precepts of palliative care. J Pall Med. 1998;1:109-12.
16. **National Hospice Organization (NHO) Standards and Accreditation Committee.** A Pathway for Patients and Families Facing Terminal Disease. Arlington, VA: NHO; 1997.
17. **Appleton M, Byock IR, Forman WB.** Academy of Hospice Physicians' position statement on access to hospice and palliative care. J Pain Symptom Manage. 1996;11:69-70.
18. **American Society of Clinical Oncology.** Cancer care during the last phase of life. J Clin Onc. 1998;16:1986-96.
19. **Coyle J, Adelhardt J, Foley K, Portenoy RK.** Character of terminal illness in the advanced cancer patient: pain and other symptoms during the last four weeks of life. J Pain Symptom Manage. 1990;5:83-93.
20. **Donnelly SM, Walsh TD.** Symptoms of advanced cancer: effects of age and gender on symptoms and survival in 1000 patients. J Palliat Care. 1994;10:91.
21. **National Hospice Organization (NHO).** Standards of a Hospice Program of Care. Arlington, VA: NHO; 1993.
22. **Cassell EJ.** Nature of suffering and the goals of medicine. N Engl J Med. 1982;306:639-41.
23. **Frank VE.** Man's Search for Meaning. New York: Washington Square Press; 1994.
24. **Byock IR.** When suffering persists. J Palliat Care. 1994;10:8-13.
25. **Adelstein DJ.** Palliative chemotherapy for non-small-cell lung cancer. Semin Oncol. 1995;22:35-9.
26. **Marino P, Pampallona S, Preatoni A, et al.** Chemotherapy vs supportive care in advanced non-small cell lung cancer: results of a meta-analysis of the literature. Chest. 1994;106:861-5.
27. **Bates T.** A review of local radiotherapy in the treatment of bone metastases and cord compression. Int J Radiation Onc Biol Phys. 1992;23:217-21.
28. **Storey P, Hill Jr HH, St Louis RH, Tarver EE.** Subcutaneous infusions for control of cancer symptoms. J Pain Symptom Manage. 1990;5:33-41.
29. **Bruera E, Roca E, Cedaro L, et al.** Action of oral methylprednisolone in terminal cancer patients: a prospective randomized double-blind study. Cancer Treatment Reports. 1985;69:751-4.

30. **Cohen SR, Mount BM.** Quality of life in terminal illness: defining and measuring subjective well-being in the dying. J Palliat Care. 1992;8:40-5.
31. **Bottomley DM, Hanks GW.** Subcutaneous midazolam infusion in palliative care. J Pain Symptom Manage. 1990;5:259-61.
32. **McNamara P, Minton M, Twycross RG.** Use of midazolam in palliative care. Palliat Med. 1991;5:244-9.
33. **Byock IR.** The nature of suffering and the nature of opportunity at the end of life. Clin Ger Med. 1996;12:237-52.
34. **Byock IR.** Dying Well. New York: Riverhead/Putnam; 1997.
35. **Butler RN.** The life review: an interpretation of reminiscence in the aged. Psychiatry. 1963;26:65-76.
36. **Stone R.** The Healing Art of Storytelling: A Sacred Journey of Personal Discovery. New York: Hyperion; 1996.
37. **Lewis MI, Butler RN.** Life-review therapy: putting memories to work in individual and group psychotherapy. Geriatrics. 1974;29:165-73.
38. **Kast V.** Joy, Inspiration, and Hope. College Station, TX: Texas A&M University Press; 1991.
39. **Fitch VT.** The psychological tasks of old age. Naropa Ins J Psychol. 1985:3:90-106.

SECTION II

Pain, Depression, Delirium, and Intractable Problems

CHAPTER 5

Management of Pain and Spinal Cord Compression in Patients with Advanced Cancer

JANET L. ABRAHM, MD

Patients with advanced cancer have substantial morbidity from moderate-to-severe pain and spinal cord compression. With appropriate multidisciplinary care, pain can be controlled in 90% of patients who have advanced malignant conditions, and 90% of ambulatory patients with spinal cord compression can remain ambulatory. Guidelines have been developed for assessing and managing patients with these problems, but implementing the guidelines can be problematic for physicians who infrequently need to use them. This chapter traces the last year of life of Mr. Simmons, a hypothetical patient who is dying of refractory prostate cancer. Mr. Simmons and his family interact with professionals from various disciplines during this year. Advance care planning is completed and activated. Practical suggestions are offered for assessment and treatment of all aspects of his pain, including its physical, psychological, social, and spiritual dimensions. The methods of pain relief used or discussed include nonpharmacologic techniques, nonopioid analgesics, opioids, adjuvant medications, radiation therapy, and radiopharmaceutical agents. Overcoming resistance to taking opioids; initiating, titrating, and changing opioid routes and agents; and preventing or relieving the side effects they induce are also covered. Data on assessment and treatment of spinal cord compression are reviewed. Physicians can use the techniques described to more readily implement existing guidelines and provide comfort and optimize quality of life for patients with advanced cancer.

Pain and spinal cord compression are two of the most distressing and disabling problems that advanced cancer patients experience. Evidence-based guidelines (1-7) and comprehensive reviews of pain assessment and pain management (8-14) show that the right combination of nonpharmacologic techniques and therapeutic agents can control pain in 85% to 95% of patients. Early recognition and treatment of spinal cord compression will preserve ambulation and continence; guidelines for management are available (15). Physicians who do not encounter many patients with moderate to severe cancer-related pain or with spinal cord compression may be unfamiliar with how to implement these guidelines in their practices. The case of Mr. Simmons, a hypothetical patient dying of refractory metastatic prostate cancer, illustrates an evidence-based approach to the most common clinical challenges such patients present.

CASE 5-1. A 72-YEAR-OLD CONSULTANT WITH PROSTATE CANCER

Mr. Simmons is a 72-year-old consultant who was found to have locally extensive prostate cancer 4 years ago. He received radiation therapy and later underwent orchiectomy and received flutamide for recurrence. The disease has become refractory to all therapies.

At the time of a routine appointment with his general internist, Mr. Simmons reports generalized aching pain "in my bones." This pain is almost always present and is exacerbated by movement. He has a history of ulcer disease. He takes acetaminophen 1000 mg four times daily. A recent bone scan revealed diffuse bony metastases in his skull, spine, hips, and femurs, with spotty involvement of his ribs. Magnetic resonance imaging showed no extension of tumor into the spinal canal. His wife reports that he is sleeping badly, is irritable, is almost confined to his recliner, and cannot attend church regularly. Mr. and Mrs. Simmons hope to join their family on a month-long cruise, and she is worried that he won't enjoy the trip.

Pain Assessment

No further diagnostic studies are needed to determine the cause of Mr. Simmons' pain; it results from his refractory metastatic prostate cancer. The functional consequences are also apparent: He is irritable, cannot sleep, and is confined to a chair. The physician should assess the intensity of the pain to determine the appropriate pharmacologic agents for initial therapy. The World Health Organization Analgesic Ladder (a repeatedly validated method for controlling pain in patients with cancer [1,2]) and the Agency for Health Care Policy and Research guidelines for treatment of cancer pain (3) recommend starting with nonopioid agents for mild pain (step 1) and adding other agents, including opioids, for moderate (step 2) or severe (step 3) pain. After therapy with pain medication is begun, repeated assessment of pain intensity enables dose adjustments in much the same way as the blood glucose level guides adjustment of the insulin dose.

Patients with chronic pain do not manifest the tachycardia, elevated blood pressure, facial grimacing, or emotional reactions typical of patients with acute pain (10). The only reliable way to determine the intensity of their pain is to ask them. Family members, physicians, and nurses regularly underestimate the intensity of pain in patients with cancer (9,16-18) or AIDS (19,20). Hispanic and black patients with cancer, elderly persons, cognitively impaired persons, women, and patients with a history of drug abuse are even more likely than other groups to have the severity of their pain underestimated and to be undertreated by physicians (16,18,20,21).

Several validated pain assessment scales (3,9) can provide an accurate measure of Mr. Simmons' pain intensity. For adults, there are three useful choices: a verbal numerical scale, a word scale (3), and visual analogue scales (Fig. 5-1). A scale that both the physician and the patient and his or her family are comfortable with should be chosen and used each time pain is reassessed. On a 0 to 10 scale, 1 to 4 represents mild pain, 5 to 6 represents moderate pain, and 7 to 10 represents severe pain.

Sitting quietly in a chair in the office and appearing tired but not in distress, Mr. Simmons surprisingly reports that his pain level is now at 9, the average intensity of his pain is 9, and his

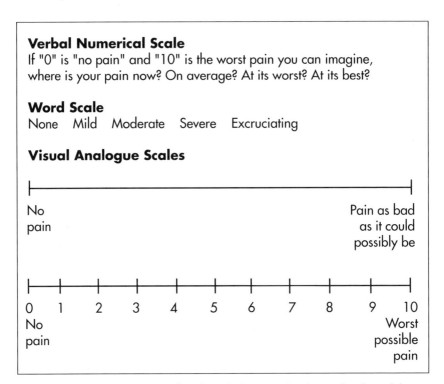

Verbal Numerical Scale
If "0" is "no pain" and "10" is the worst pain you can imagine, where is your pain now? On average? At its worst? At its best?

Word Scale
None   Mild   Moderate   Severe   Excruciating

Visual Analogue Scales

No pain   Pain as bad
                                                as it could
                                                possibly be

0   1   2   3   4   5   6   7   8   9   10
No   Worst
pain   possible
                                                pain

Figure 5-1. Pain assessment scales. The verbal numerical scale, word scale, and the two visual analogue scales shown are four validated, commonly used scales for pain assessment. On a visual analogue scale, the patient marks the point that represents the intensity of his or her pain now, on average, at its worst, and at its best. See Reference 3 for more information.

*worst pain is at least 10. For a few hours after he takes aceta-
minophen, his pain level falls to 8.*

Therapy for Bone Pain

Mr. Simmons' bone pain is too diffuse for standard radiation of the most painful metastases. In this case, because none of the remedies discussed below is curative and each has different risks, benefits, and costs, the patient's preferences should be sought before one is chosen.

Pharmacologic Therapy

Adjuvant therapy with acetaminophen can be continued (3,22). Considering Mr. Simmons' age and ulcer history, nonsteroidal anti-inflammatory drugs (NSAIDs), which inhibit both COX-1 and COX-2, would not ordinarily be included in his initial regimen. They have a high incidence of inducing gastrointestinal toxicity in this population (22-25). If an NSAID is added, misoprostol (200 μg qid) or omeprazole (20 mg qd) are also indicated (26,27).

The mainstay of therapy for severe pain is a step 3 opioid (3,28-42) (Table 5-1) and a laxative (2,43-45) (Fig. 5-2). When opioids are used in pain management, the following should be done:

1. Use the World Health Organization analgesic ladder. Advance up the ladder if pain persists.
2. Prescribe drug doses high enough to relieve the pain and administer the drugs frequently enough to prevent recurrence of pain (3-5,11).
3. Provide a "rescue" dose of a short-acting opioid for unexpected pain exacerbations (3,46). This dose should be 10% of the total daily opioid dose (13). Sustained-release preparations of oxycodone or morphine, as well as transdermal fentanyl (47,48), can be used to control continuous baseline pain. Transdermal fentanyl diffuses into a skin reservoir from which it enters the bloodstream (33). There is, therefore, a 12-hour to 24-hour delay in onset of pain relief and, should toxicity occur, a similar delay in its resolution (49). Because of this, immediate-release opioids are routinely required for opioid-naive patients in whom therapy with transdermal fentanyl is begun (33).

The physician should also prescribe immediate-release opioids at this time to treat unexpected exacerbations of pain or pain that occurs only with movement. These rescue doses (3,46) of morphine, oxycodone, or hydromorphone start at 10% of the total daily opioid dose and are given every 1 to 2 hr as needed (13). The dose of the oral transmucosal fentanyl lozenge must be individually determined (38-42).

Meperidine is not indicated for repeated dosing in patients with chronic severe pain (3,8). It has poor oral bioavailability and a short therapeutic half-life. Toxic levels of its metabolite, normeperidine,

Table 5-1. Opioids for Step 3 (Severe) Pain.*

Opioid	Initial Dose (mg)†		Dose Interval (h)	Preparations
	Oral	Parenteral		
Morphine				
Immediate release	15–30	10	3–4	Intravenous, intramuscular, subcutaneous, tablet, rectal, liquid, liquid concentrate
Sustained release	30–60	NA	8–12	Tablet
Sustained release	60–120	NA	12–24	Capsule with pellets
Hydromorphone (immediate release)	6	1.5	3–4	Intravenous, intramuscular, subcutaneous, tablet, rectal
Oxycodone plus level 1 agents	10	NA	3–4	Tablet, liquid
Oxycodone	10–20	NA	3–4	Tablet, liquid, liquid concentrate
Oxycodone (sustained release)	30–60	NA	12	Tablet
Fentanyl	NA	50‡	72	Transdermal
	200‡	NA	4	Transmucosal oralet
Methadone	20	10	6–8	Intramuscular, intravenous, subcutaneous§, tablet, liquid
Meperidine¶	300	100	3	Intramuscular, intravenous, tablet

* Data from References 3, 28–30, 32, 33, 36–42. NA = not applicable.
† For patients weighing more than 110 lb who have moderate to severe pain. Initial doses should be halved for opioid-naive patients, elderly persons, or medically frail persons. Data from Management of Cancer Pain; Adults AHCPR 94-0592.
‡ Values given are µg/h.
§ Least recommended route; pain and pruritus often develop at the infusion site.
¶ Not recommended for patients with advanced cancer.

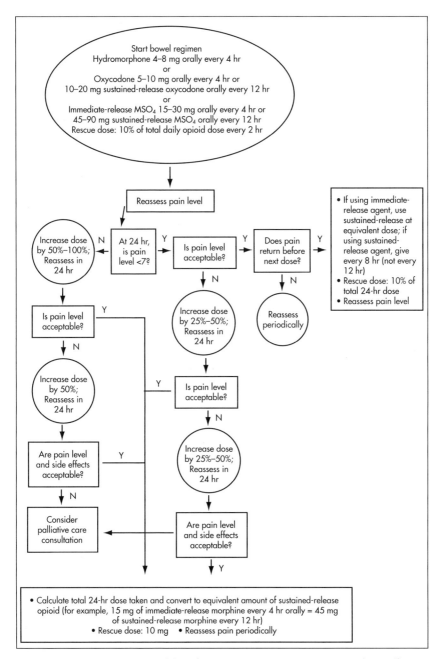

Figure 5-2. Management guidelines for severe cancer pain. MSO$_4$ = morphine sulfate.

accumulate with repeated dosing or in patients with renal insufficiency and can cause dysphoria, myoclonic jerks, and seizures (50).

Nonpharmacologic Therapy

Nonpharmacologic therapies are very useful adjuncts to pharmacologic therapy in addressing even severe cancer pain. A variety of physical and cognitive techniques can diminish Mr. Simmons' experience of pain (49-57). Physiatrists and physical and occupational therapists can recommend positions to maximize his comfort and offer advice regarding exercise and assist devices (e.g., lift chairs or a trapeze over his bed) to maximize his mobility (50,51). He or his wife can apply heat to the area of bone discomfort, and he can receive massages to diminish muscle spasm (49,50,52), or he can try acupuncture therapy, although it has not been extensively studied in patients like Mr. Simmons. Transcutaneous electrical nerve stimulation is less likely to be helpful because it is most effective with pain that is in a dermatomal distribution (49).

Both progressive muscle relaxation (53,54) and hypnosis (55), however, have been shown in controlled trials to decrease cancer pain (53,55). Using hypnosis, Mr. Simmons can learn to dissociate or distract himself from the pain, and both techniques induce deep relaxation that improves sleep and decreases muscle tension. Screening for psychological, social, or spiritual concerns that are exacerbating his experience of pain should be offered (54). Spiritual or psychological counseling, with or without hypnosis, might be valuable if he needs help developing coping skills or if the screening reveals spiritual concerns, untreated anxiety or depression, or a history of coping poorly in the past (56,57).

Other Therapeutic Options

Bone pain can also be relieved by bisphosphonates or by radiation delivered by radiopharmaceuticals or by external beam. The bisphosphonates have shown impressive pain relieving activity in patients with lytic metastases from multiple myeloma and breast cancer (58-62). However, although they have been effective in small trials of patients with prostate cancer (63), no large-scale double-blind trials have been completed to assess their efficacy in patients with blastic bone disease. Phase III trials are currently underway (60).

Nuclear medicine specialists administer the radiopharmaceuticals strontium-89 (64-67), rhenium-186 HEDP (65), and samarium-153 lexidronam (68-70) to relieve the pain of blastic metastases. Phase III double-blind placebo-controlled trials of rhenium are underway (65) and those of both samarium (68) and ^{89}Sr documented their effectiveness. By far, most trials have been conducted using ^{89}Sr. Strontium-89 is a pure beta-emitter that incorporates into bone in areas of osteoblastic activity adjacent to metastases but not into normal bone or marrow or metastases where there is no blastic activity, as in multiple myeloma (64,65,67,71). Pain relief begins in 1 to 2 weeks. It is complete in 10% to 30% of patients, and pain is significantly improved in 80% with a median response duration of 3 to 6 months (64,65). Safety of repeated dosing has not been extensively studied but up to 10 doses have been given in 3-month intervals without incident (65).

Five percent to 10% of patients will suffer a "flare" (i.e., an increase in bone pain) 2 to 3 days after the injection. Flares are more common in cancer of the breast than of the prostate (72,73). Myelosuppression occurs in most patients with drops of platelet and leukocyte counts of 25% to 40%. Strontium-89 is therefore contraindicated in patients with a platelet count of <60,000/mm^3 or leukocytes of <2400/mm^3 (65). Initial blood counts and previous irradiation of marrow do not predict the extent of the subsequent reductions in blood counts (64). Life-threatening thrombocytopenia, however, has been noted in patients with low-grade disseminated intravascular coagulation or rapidly failing platelet counts (74).

Mr. Simmons also could be evaluated by the radiation oncologist for hemibody radiation, which relieves pain from metastases in the lower spine, pelvis, and femora (64) in as many as 80% of prostate cancer patients, with 30% obtaining complete relief. The relief begins as early as 48 hours after treatment (75) and lasts a median of 4 to 8.5 months, depending on how the radiation is delivered (76). Hemibody radiation is not often chosen as initial therapy for patients with bony metastases because of technical difficulties in delivering the radiation and concerns about side effects and toxicity to viscera and bone marrow that exceed those of radiopharmaceuticals (64,67).

Mr. Simmons' physician presents Mr. and Mrs. Simmons with what she feels are the best initial options: opioid therapy and nonpharmacologic methods. They accept lift and bath chairs and a new heating pad. They have begun regular discussions with their pastor and feel that he provides adequate psychological support. But Mr. Simmons refuses the opioid prescription.

Patient Reluctance To Take Opioids

Like many other patients with cancer, Mr. Simmons probably harbors numerous misconceptions about opioids: fear of becoming an addict, "feeling high," using up the effective agents and having nothing left if the pain gets worse, and developing refractory constipation (3,14). To explore patient fears and enhance compliance, physicians must help him understand several aspects of opioid use. First, there is a distinction between tolerance, physical dependence, and psychological addiction. Second, the chances of addiction are less than 1% (72-75). Third, patients will not "feel high" on effective doses of opioids; moreover, a feeling of euphoria does not imply that the patient is misusing the medication. Finally, even if the patient takes medication now, he will still be able to achieve pain relief by using higher doses if the pain worsens.

Constipation, the most common opioid-induced side effect, usually does not resolve with time (11,43-45,75), but daily laxatives prevent or at least improve opioid-induced constipation (11,44,75,76). The most effective agents are senna (1 or 2 tablets, once or twice daily; the dose can be increased as needed), senna combined with a stool softener, bisacodyl, milk of magnesia alone or with mineral oil, and lactulose (1 to 2 tablespoons at bedtime; the dose can be increased as needed). Lactulose is the most expensive of these treatments (76). In selected patients, 1 tablespoon of polyethylene glycol in 4 oz of water may be needed. Fiber intake should not be increased because, as patients become more debilitated, fiber is more likely to exacerbate than to relieve the problem (75). Once a stable dose of opioid is reached, nausea and sedation will resolve and the patient will be able to participate in usual activities including driving (77).

Mr. Simmons admits that, for him, accepting opioids means accepting death. He was also concerned about retaining his mental clarity and about what his children might think when they learned that he was "taking dope." Following his pastor's advice, however, he spoke with his children, and they alleviated these concerns.

Mr. Simmons' pain is relieved by 30 mg of immediate-release morphine every 4 hr, and his therapy is switched to the equivalent dose of sustained-release morphine (90 mg every 12 hr) plus rescue doses of 15 mg of immediate-release morphine every 2 hr as needed; an equivalent is 60 mg of controlled-release oxycodone plus rescue doses of 10 mg of immediate-release oxycodone (see Appendix) (3,36,78). Senna (2 tablets twice daily) is added to Mr. Simmons' regimen, and prochlorperazine is available for nausea. Mr. Simmons mentions feeling mildly sedated, but his physician tells him that this effect will probably resolve by the end of the week.

Two days later, Mr. Simmons reports that with his increased activity he needed six rescue doses (90 mg) of morphine each day to maintain an average pain level of 6. He felt that this was too high.

Titrating an Opioid-Containing Regimen

Mr. Simmons took more than 25% of his daily scheduled morphine as rescue doses, which suggests that he needs a higher regularly scheduled morphine dose. Despite the rescue doses, his pain level remains moderate (level of 5 to 6); thus he requires a 25% higher total daily morphine dose (see Fig. 5-2).

Mr. Simmons begins therapy with sustained-release morphine 160 mg every 12 hr plus rescue doses of immediate-release morphine 30 mg (Appendix, Titration). Twenty-four hours later, his pain level is 3, which is acceptable. He slept through the night and ambulates comfortably. He confides that when the pain was at its worst, he began to wonder what he had done to cause God to abandon him. Despite reassurances from his pastor, he felt a growing sense of despair and isolation from his family and his faith that began to resolve when he resumed attending Sunday church services.

*Three days later, Mr. Simmons' pain is still well con-
trolled, but he has developed significant nausea that is unresponsive to oral prochlorperazine 10 mg 3 times daily. He is
not constipated, and the nausea is not positional or precipi-
tated by the sight or smell of food. It is exacerbated by a rescue
dose of immediate-release morphine.*

Therapy for Opioid-Induced Nausea

Mr. Simmons has not been receiving chemotherapy, and he has no evidence of vertigo, gastroparesis, or bowel obstruction (79-81). Morphine
is the probable cause of his nausea, and changing from morphine to
another opioid may eliminate it (82,83); conversion techniques are
described in the Appendix. Sustained-release oxycodone and transdermal fentanyl are easier to use but more expensive than equianalgesic
doses of methadone (76,84-86).

*Mr. Simmons refuses methadone therapy because "it's a drug
for addicts" and refuses transdermal fentanyl because it is too
visible. Therapy with sustained-release oxycodone 70 mg every
12 hr (330 mg of sustained-release morphine = 220 mg sustained-release oxycodone; two-thirds of 220 mg of sustained-
release oxycodone = 145 mg over 24 hr) is therefore started
(Appendix, Conversion). Three days later, he is no longer nauseated, and his pain level remains at 3; exacerbations are controlled by 15 mg of immediate-release oxycodone (10% of 140
mg = about 15 mg). He has no new adverse effects.*

*A week later, Mr. and Mrs. Simmons leave on their cruise,
which turns out to be all they had hoped for. A month later,
however, Mr. Simmons' pain with movement has increased
and he feels too sedated from the frequent oxycodone rescue
doses. He accepts treatment with ^{89}Sr. Three weeks later, Mrs.
Simmons reports that her husband is much more nauseated
and somnolent. He has no pain at rest and has minimal pain
when he changes position, and he has needed no rescue opioids. Laboratory studies show normal levels of electrolytes, calcium, and albumin and normal renal and hepatic function.*

Treatment of Opioid-Induced Sedation

Mr. Simmons' opioid-induced sedation and nausea have most likely re-emerged because therapy with ^{89}Sr decreased his bone pain. Naloxone is not needed to reverse these effects. Decreasing the oxycodone dose by approximately 50% (to 40 mg of sustained-release oxycodone every 12 hr plus 10-mg rescue doses) should alleviate the sedation. Naloxone would precipitate symptoms of opioid withdrawal (87) and reverse analgesia. If significant respiratory depression occurs (88), appropriate therapy would be just enough of the standard 0.4 mg of naloxone diluted in 10 mL of saline to reverse the respiratory depression (3).

> *Mr. Simmons' oxycodone dose is reduced as recommended, and within 36 hr he is again alert, does not have nausea, and has an average pain level of 3, which is acceptable to him.*
>
> *Three months later, Mr. Simmons visits the emergency department because of increasing discomfort in his mid-back region, with pain radiating to his right nipple. Comprehensive neurologic examination reveals normal finding, and no herpetic lesions are visible. Plain radiographs of the spine show diffuse blastic metastatic disease that includes the area of the pain. The dose of oral sustained-release oxycodone is increased to 60 mg every 12 hr, with a rescue dose of 10 mg. The next day, Mr. Simmons' back pain is at a level of 3 to 4. He continues to have normal bowel movements.*

Assessment of Back Pain in Patients with Cancer

Mr. Simmons has thoracic spine pain, radiculopathy, and evidence on plain radiographs of metastatic disease in the area of his pain, a location typical for metastatic prostate cancer (89). There is a 90% probability that the prostate cancer has spread to the epidural space and that the spinal cord is in jeopardy (90-93). Even without the radiculopathy, the probability of epidural disease would be 60% to 70% (90-92). Normal findings on physical examination do not diminish this probability.

If a patient is treated while he or she is still ambulatory, the probability of remaining ambulatory is 89% to 94% (15,67,94-96). If a patient becomes paraparetic before therapy, the probability of regaining the ability to ambulate is only 39% to 51%; if he or she becomes paralyzed, it decreases to 10% (15,67,95). Emergency magnetic resonance imaging of the entire spine is probably preferable to CT myelography, which is potentially associated with more complications (95) and is no more sensitive or specific (89,94).

> *Mr. Simmons undergoes MRI of the spine, which reveals metastases to multiple thoracic vertebrae and epidural spread with early cord compression at T6.*

Corticosteroid Therapy for Malignant Spinal Cord Compression

Corticosteroid therapy decreases cord edema (97) and pain, helps preserve neurologic function, and improves overall outcome after specific therapy (98). High-dose dexamethasone (100 mg intravenous bolus followed by 24 mg orally 4 times daily for 3 days, then tapered over 10 days) is probably indicated for patients with impaired function of the spinal cord or cauda equina or with a high-grade radiologic lesion. At this dose, the drug substantially increases the number of these patients who remain ambulatory (81% compared with 63%) (98). Other patients usually receive lower-dose regimens (10 mg intravenous bolus followed by 4 mg intravenously 4 times daily, then tapered over 14 days); these are better tolerated (15) but may not improve the patient's chance of remaining ambulatory (57.1% compared with 57.9%) (99).

Radiation Therapy with or without Surgery

Surgical decompression is advocated to establish the diagnosis (15); to treat a single site of suspected involvement (15); to treat progression despite radiation therapy (100); or to treat vertebral instability, collapse with bone impinging on the spinal cord, or displacement (15).

Surgery is not advocated for metastases from prostate or breast cancer, myeloma, or lymphoma, which are likely (70% to 88%) to respond to radiation therapy (95,96). Back pain will resolve in 70% to

85% of cases (94,95). Ambulatory patients are equally likely to remain ambulatory with radiation therapy or surgery (101-103).

> *Mr. Simmons agrees to radiation therapy and corticosteroids because he hopes to "dance with my bride" at his 50th anniversary party. Three weeks later, further discussion with the Simmons family about their hopes, goals, and the burdens and benefits of hospitalization lead to enrollment in hospice care, although Mr. Simmons still wishes to be resuscitated.*
>
> *Mrs. Simmons later reports that the hospice team has markedly decreased her anxiety. An experienced nurse now evaluates her husband frequently; their eldest daughter agreed to be Mr. Simmons' health care proxy and, on the social worker's recommendation, the necessary financial and funeral arrangements have been made.*
>
> *Mr. Simmons responds well to therapy, but over the next 6 weeks his oral opioid requirements reach 100 mg of sustained-release oxycodone every 12 hr and he is more sedated. Repeated laboratory testing reveals no contributing metabolic abnormalities. Psychiatric evaluation fails to detect evidence of depression. His anniversary party is only 1 week away, and he wants to be "sharp" then.*

Further Treatment of Opioid-Induced Sedation

For patients in Mr. Simmons' circumstance, changing the adjuvant acetaminophen therapy to treatment with a nonsteroidal anti-inflammatory drug might allow the opioid dose to be reduced without sacrificing pain control. If this is insufficient, adding a psychostimulant without decreasing the opioid dose is likely to increase alertness (in Mr. Simmons' case, in time for him to enjoy the party) (104-107). Effective agents include methylphenidate or dextroamphetamine (initial dose: 2.5 to 5 mg orally in the morning and repeated at noon if necessary) and pemoline, a chewable tablet (initial dose: 18.75 mg orally in the morning and repeated at noon) that is more expensive (76). Doses should be increased as needed. The patient might also be referred for instruction in hypnosis or relaxation techniques.

Mr. Simmons declines referral for hypnosis and relaxation instruction and is unable to tolerate the gastrointestinal side effects of low-dose ibuprofen. Therefore he begins taking methylphenidate 2.5 mg at 8 a.m. and noon. Three days later, without a change in opioid dose, he reports feeling "back to normal." After the party, Mr. Simmons' daughter calls the office to thank the physician for helping her parents fully enjoy their anniversary celebration.

Two weeks later, Mr. Simmons' pain again increases. When the physician visits their home, the pastor is present on one of his almost daily visits. He participates in the discussion with the Simmons family, in which Mr. Simmons reiterates his desire to die at home and states that he does not want resuscitation. Mr. Simmons asks the physician to limit his medications to pain relievers and laxatives. Over the next few weeks, he becomes less interactive, stays in bed more of the day, and asks for food less often. A hospice home health aide helps Mrs. Simmons with his care 2 hr a day, and hospice volunteers sit with him while Mrs. Simmons does her marketing. A harpist who is a music therapist visits several times a week. Because of his decreased activity, Mr. Simmons now requires a sustained-release oxycodone dose of 160 mg every 12 hr.

When Mr. Simmons is closer to death and unable to swallow pills, his family is offered the choice of giving him hourly sublingual liquid oxycodone concentrate (0.66 mL of a 20 mg/mL solution each hour; 320 mg of sustained-release oxycodone = 320 mg of immediate-release oxycodone in 24 hr; 320 mg of 20 mg/mL = 16 mL in 24 hr) or a subcutaneous opioid infusion. Because they are unsure that he will remain comfortable while receiving the liquid opioid, the family requests an opioid infusion. Hydromorphone is chosen to minimize the amount of subcutaneous fluid required (see Appendix). Mr. Simmons dies peacefully the next day.

Summary

Although treatments vary in efficacy, similar approaches are available for the other physical and mental disorders that afflict patients like Mr.

Simmons. The roles of the health care team, social workers, and spiritual advisors, and the management strategies for fatigue, weakness, xerostomia, delirium, anxiety, depression, anorexia, and decubiti are reviewed in several recent textbooks (108-111), handbooks (112,113), a case-based manual (114), and a resource document (115). With these resources and the information supplied by hospice and palliative care teams, general internists can relieve much of the distress in patients with advanced cancer.

Appendix

Believe the Patient's Report of Pain

1. To assess and manage the patient's pain, use a pain scale.
2. For mild pain (1 to 4 on a 0 to 10 scale), start with aspirin, acetaminophen, or a nonsteroidal anti-inflammatory drug.
3. If the pain is not relieved or is moderate (pain score: 5 to 6), add oxycodone, tramadol, or hydrocodone (or use a combination product that contains 5 mg oxycodone or hydrocodone with aspirin, acetaminophen, or a nonsteroidal anti-inflammatory drug).
4. For severe pain (pain score: 7 to 10), start therapy with oxycodone alone, hydromorphone, or morphine. If a transdermal opioid is desired, consider using transdermal fentanyl after the effective opioid dose has been identified by using immediate-release agents.
5. Transdermal fentanyl has a 14- to 24-hr "on-and-off" time.
6. If the pain is excruciating (pain score >10), increase the opioid dose by 50% to 100%, regardless of the amount of drug given, until the pain is relieved.
7. For chronic pain, give around-the-clock therapy or "patient may refuse," not "as-needed therapy."
8. For pain between doses, give 10% of the total daily opioid dose in immediate-release form (e.g., the rescue dose for 200 mg opioid is 20 mg).
9. Always prescribe a laxative (such as senna with or without lactulose); do not give "as needed." Patient may need an antiemetic for 2 to 7 days.
10. Avoid benzodiazepine sleep medications.

Opioid Dose Titration

- Current total dose = (90 mg every 12 hr) + rescue dose (15 mg × 6) = 180 mg + 90 mg = 270 mg
- Calculated new total dose = (270 mg) + (270 mg × 25% = 67.5 mg) = 337.5 mg
- Relevant available sustained-release morphine doses are 15, 30, 60, and 100 mg
- Actual new regimen = 160 mg every 12 hr to 175 mg every 12 hr, plus a 30-mg rescue dose

Opioid Conversion

Determine the equianalgesic dose of the new opioid (Table 5-2) and prescribe two thirds of this dose to allow for incomplete cross-tolerance.

Table 5-3 gives the equianalgesic doses of fentanyl and morphine. Prescribe the full doses (data are from direct *in vivo* comparisons).

Acknowledgements

The author thanks Dr. Daniel Haller, the members of the ACP-ASIM End-of-Life Care Consensus Panel, and the outside reviewers for critiquing the manuscript. The Open Society Institute Project on Death in America Faculty Scholars Program provided salary support. The opinions expressed here are those of the author and not necessarily those of the Open Society Institute.

Table 5-2.   Opioid Equianalgesic Doses.*

Drug	Oral (mg)	Parenteral (mg)
Morphine	30	10
Hydromorphone	7.5	1.5
Oxycodone	20	NA
Levorphanol	4	2
Meperidine[†]	300	100

* Data from References 3, 36, 37, 78.
[†] Not recommended.
NA = not applicable.

Table 5-3. Equianalgesic Doses of Fentanyl and Morphine.

Fentanyl (µg/h)	Morphine (mg/24h)*	
	Oral	Parenteral
25	30–90	10–30
50	91–150	31–50
75	151–210	51–70
100	211–270	71–90
125	271–330	91–110
150	331–390	111–130
200	451–510	151–170

* Data from Reference 35.

REFERENCES

1. **Zech DF, Grond S, Lynch J, et al.** Validation of World Health Organization Guidelines for cancer pain relief: a 10-year prospective study. Pain. 1995;63:65-76.
2. Cancer Pain Relief: With a Guide to Opioid Availability. 2nd ed. Geneva: World Health Organization; 1996.
3. **Jacox A, Carr DB, Payne R, et al.** Management of Cancer Pain. Clinical Practice Guideline No. 9. Rockville, MD: U.S. Department of Health and Human Services, Public Health Service, Agency for Health Care Policy and Research; 1994; ACHPR Publication No. 94-0592.
4. Cancer Pain Assessment and Treatment Curriculum Guidelines. The Ad Hoc Committee on Cancer Pain of the American Society of Clinical Oncology. J Clin Oncol. 1992;10:1976-82.
5. Principles of Analgesic Use in the Treatment of Acute Pain and Cancer Pain. Skokie, IL: American Pain Society; 1992.
6. Practice Guidelines for Cancer Pain Management. A report by the American Society of Anesthesiologists Task Force on Pain Management, Cancer Pain Section. Anesthesiology. 1996;84:1243-57.
7. **American Geriatrics Society.** The management of chronic pain in older persons: AGS Panel on Chronic Pain in Older Persons. J Am Geriatr Soc. 1998;46:635-51.
8. **Foley KM.** Management of cancer pain. In: DeVita VT, Hellman S, Rosenberg SA, Eds. Cancer: Principles and Practice of Oncology. 5th ed. Philadelphia: Lippincott-Raven; 1997:2807-41.
9. **Ingham J, Portenoy RK.** The measurement of pain and other symptoms. In: Doyle D, Hanks GW, MacDonald N, Eds. Oxford Textbook of Palliative Medicine. 2d ed. Oxford: Oxford University Press; 1997:203-19.

10. **McGuire DB.** The multiple dimensions of cancer pain: a framework for assessment and management. In: McGuire DB, Yarbro CH, Ferrell BR, Eds. Cancer Pain Management. 2nd ed. Boston: Jones and Bartlett; 1995:1-17.

11. **Levy MH.** Pharmacologic treatment of cancer pain. N Engl J Med. 1996;335:1124-32.

12. **Cherny NI, Foley KM.** Pain and Palliative Care. Hematol Oncol Clin North Am. Volume 10. Philadelphia: WB Saunders; 1996.

13. **Cherny NI, Portenoy RK.** Cancer pain management: current strategy. Cancer. 1993;72(11 Suppl):3393-415.

14. **Foley KM.** Pain assessment and cancer pain syndromes. In: Doyle D, Hanks GW, MacDonald N, Eds. Oxford Textbook of Palliative Medicine. 2nd ed. Oxford: Oxford University Press; 1997:310-31.

15. **Loblaw DA, Laperierre NJ.** Emergency treatment of malignant extradural spinal cord compression: an evidence-based guideline. J Clin Oncol. 1998;16:1613-24.

16. **Cleeland CS, Gonin R, Hatfield AK, et al.** Pain and its treatment in outpatients with metastatic cancer. N Engl J Med. 1994;330:592-6.

17. **Grossman SA, Sheidler VR, Swedeen K, et al.** Correlation of patient and caregiver ratings of cancer pain. J Pain Symptom Manage. 1991;6:53-7.

18. **Cleeland CS, Gonin R, Baez L, et al.** Pain and treatment of pain in minority patients with cancer. The Eastern Cooperative Oncology Group Minority Outpatient Pain Study. Ann Intern Med. 1997;127:813-6.

19. **Breitbart W, Rosenfeld BD, Passik SD, et al.** The undertreatment of pain in ambulatory AIDS patients. Pain. 1996;65:243-9.

20. **Breitbart W, Rosenfeld B, Passik S, et al.** A comparison of pain report and adequacy of analgesic therapy in ambulatory AIDS patients with and without a history of substance abuse. Pain. 1997;72:235-43.

21. **Ferrell BA, Ferrell BR, Rivera L.** Pain in cognitively impaired nursing home patients. J Pain Symptom Manage. 1995;10:591-8.

22. **Eisenberg E, Berkey CS, Carr DB, et al.** Efficacy and safety of non-steroidal antiinflammatory drugs for cancer pain: a meta-analysis. J Clin Oncol. 1994;12:2756-65.

23. **Gloth FM, III.** Concerns with chronic analgesic therapy in elderly patients. Am J Med. 1996;101(Suppl 1):19S-24S.

24. **Ferrell BA.** Pain evaluation and management in the nursing home. Ann Intern Med. 1995;123:681-7.

25. **Roth SH.** Merits and liabilities of NSAID therapy. Rheum Dis Clin North Am. 1989;15:479-98.

26. **Hawkey CJ, Karrasch KA, Szczepanski L, et al.** Omeprazole compared with misoprostol for ulcers associated with nonsteroidal antiinflammatory drugs. Omeprazole versus Misoprostol for NSAID-Induced Ulcer Management (OMNIUM) Study Group. N Engl J Med. 1998;338:727-34.

27. **Yeomans ND, Tulassay Z, Juhasz L, et al.** A comparison of omeprazole with ranitidine for ulcers associated with nonsteroidal antiinflammatory

drugs. Acid Suppression Trial: Ranitidine versus Omeprazole for NSAID-Associated Ulcer Treatment (ASTRONAUT) Study Group. N Engl J Med. 1998;338:719-26.

28. **Westerling D, Lindahl S, Andersson KE, Andersson A.** Absorption and bioavailability of rectally administered morphine in women. Eur J Clin Pharmacol. 1982;23:59-64.

29. **De Conno F, Ripamonti C, Saiti L, et al.** Role of rectal route in treating cancer pain: a randomized crossover clinical trial of oral versus rectal morphine administration in opioid-naive cancer patients with pain. J Clin Oncol. 1995;13:1004-8.

30. **Kaiko R, Lacouture P, Hopf K, et al.** Analgesic onset and potency of oral controlled-release (CR) oxycodone and CR morphine [Abstract]. Clin Pharmacol Ther. 1996;59:130.

31. **Bruera ED, Chadwick S, Bacovsky R, MacDonald N.** Continuous subcutaneous infusion of narcotics using a portable disposable pump. J Palliat Care. 1985;1:46-7.

32. **Broomhead A, West R, Knox K, et al.** Morphine bioavailability and pharmacokinetic comparison of Kadian (sustained release morphine sulfate) capsules and pellets ("sprinkling") in human volunteers under fasted or fed conditions [Abstact]. Proc Am Soc Clin Oncol. 1997;16:61a.

33. **Varvel JR, Shafer SL, Hwang SS, et al.** Absorption characteristics of transdermally administered fentanyl. Anesthesiology. 1989;70:928-34.

34. **Portenoy RK, Southam MA, Gupta SK, et al.** Transdermal fentanyl for cancer pain: repeated dose pharmacokinetics. Anesthesiology. 1993;78:36-43.

35. **Donner B, Zenz M, Tryba M, Strumpf M.** Direct conversion from oral morphine to transdermal fentanyl: a multicenter study in patients with cancer pain. Pain. 1996;64:527-34.

36. **Hanks GW, Cherny N.** Opioid analgesic therapy. In: Doyle D, Hanks GW, MacDonald N, Eds. Oxford Textbook of Palliative Medicine. 2nd ed. Oxford: Oxford University Press; 1997:351-5.

37. **Kaplan R, Parris WC, Citron ML, et al.** Comparison of controlled-release and immediate-release oxycodone tablets in patients with cancer pain. J Clin Oncol. 1998;16:3230-7.

38. **Fine PG, Marcus M, De Boer AJ, Van der Oord B.** An open-label study of oral transmucosal fentanyl citrate (OTFC) for the treatment of breakthrough cancer pain. Pain. 1991;45:149-53.

39. **Streisand JB, Varvel JR, Stanski DR, et al.** Absorption and bioavailability of oral transmucosal fentanyl citrate. Anesthesiology. 1991;75:223-9.

40. **Christie JM, Simmonds MA, Patt R, et al.** Dose-titration, multicenter study of oral transmucosal fentanyl citrate for the treatment of breakthrough pain in cancer patients using transdermal fentanyl for persistent pain. J Clin Oncol. 1998;16:3238-45.

41. **Lyss AP.** Long-term use of oral transmucosal fentanyl citrate (OTFC) for breakthrough pain in cancer patients [Abstract]. Proc ASCO. 1997;16:41a.

42. **Farrar JT, Cleary J, Rauck R, et al.** Oral transmucosal fentanyl citrate: randomized, double-blinded, placebo-controlled trial for treatment of breakthrough pain in cancer patients. J Natl Cancer Inst. 1998;90:611-6.

43. **Bruera E, Suarez-Almazor M, Velasco A, et al.** The assessment of constipation in terminal cancer patients admitted to a palliative care unit: a retrospective review. J Pain Symptom Manage. 1994;9:515-9.

44. **Glare P, Lickiss JN.** Unrecognized constipation in patients with advanced cancer: a recipe for disaster. J Pain Symptom Manage. 1992;7:369-71.

45. **Billings JA.** Outpatient Management of Advanced Cancer: Symptom Control, Support, and Hospice in-the-Home. Philadelphia: Lippincott; 1985:69-76.

46. **Patt RB, Ellison NM.** Breakthrough pain in cancer patients: characteristics, prevalence, and treatment. Oncology (Huntingt). 1998;12:1035-46.

47. **Ahmedzai S, Brooks D.** Transdermal fentanyl versus sustained-release oral morphine in cancer pain: preference, efficacy, and quality of life. The TTS-Fentanyl Comparative Trial Group. J Pain Symptom Manage. 1997;13:254-61.

48. **Payne R, Mathias SD, Pasta DJ, et al.** Quality of life and cancer pain: satisfaction and side effects with transdermal fentanyl versus oral morphine. J Clin Oncol. 1998;16:1588-93.

49. **Coyle N, Cherny N, Portenoy RK.** Pharmacologic management of cancer pain. In: McGuire DB, Yarbro CH, Ferrell BR, Eds. Cancer Pain Management. 2nd ed. Boston: Jones and Bartlett; 1995:89-130.

50. **Kaiko RF, Foley KM, Grabinski PY, et al.** Central nervous system excitatory effects of meperidine in cancer patients. Ann Neurol. 1983;13:180-5.

51. **Spross JA, Wolff Burke M.** Nonpharmacologic management of cancer pain. In: McGuire DB, Yarbro CH, Ferrell BR, Eds. Cancer Pain Management. 2nd ed. Boston: Jones and Bartlett; 1995:159-205.

52. **Rhiner M, Ferrell BR, Ferrell BA, Grant MM.** A structured nondrug intervention program for cancer pain. Cancer Pract. 1993;1:137-43.

53. **McCaffery M, Wolff M.** Pain relief using cutaneous modalities, positioning, and movement. Hosp J. 1992;8:121-54.

54. **Ferrell-Torry A, Glick O.** The use of therapeutic massage as a nursing intervention to modify anxiety and the perception of cancer pain. Cancer Nurs. 1993;16:93-101.

55. **Syrjala KL, Donaldson GW, Davis MW, et al.** Relaxation and imagery and cognitive-behavioral training reduce pain during cancer treatment: a controlled clinical trial. Pain. 1995;63:189-98.

56. **Benson H, Beary JF, Carol MP.** The relaxation response. Psychiatry. 1974;37:37-46.

57. **Syrjala KL, Roth-Roemer SL.** Hypnosis and suggestion for managing cancer pain. In: Barber J, Ed. Hypnosis and Suggestion in the Treatment of Pain. New York: WW Norton; 1996:121-57.

58. **Loscalzo M.** Psychological approaches to the management of pain in patients with advanced cancer. Hematol Oncol Clin North Am. 1996;10:139-55.

59. **Breitbart W, Passik SD, Rosenfeld BD.** Psychiatric and psychological aspects of cancer pain. In: Wall PD, Melzack R, Eds. Textbook of Pain. 3rd ed. New York: Churchill Livingstone; 1994:825-59.
60. **Hortobagyi GN, Theriault RL, Porter L, et al.** Efficacy of pamidronate in reducing skeletal complications in patients with breast cancer and lytic bone metastases. Protocol 19 Aredia Breast Cancer Study Group. N Engl J Med. 1996;335:1785-91.
61. **Hortobagyi GN, Theriault RL, Lipton A, et al.** Long-term prevention of skeletal complications of metastatic breast cancer with pamidronate. Protocol 19 Aredia Breast Cancer Study Group. J Clin Oncol. 1998;16:2038-44.
62. **Lipton A.** Bisphosphonates treatment of lytic bone metastases. ASCO Education Book, Spring 1998. Philadelphia: WB Saunders; 1998:94-9.
63. **Coleman RE, Purohilt OP, Vinholes JJ, Zekri J.** High dose pamidronate: clinical and biochemical effects in metastatic bone disease. Cancer. 1997;80:1686-90.
64. **Berenson JR, Lichtenstein A, Porter L, et al.** Long-term pamidronate treatment of advanced multiple myeloma patients reduces skeletal events. J Clin Oncol. 1998;16:593-602.
65. **Adami S.** Bisphosphonates in prostate carcinoma. Cancer. 1997;80(8 Suppl):1674-9.
66. **Robinson RG, Preston DF, Baxter KG, et al.** Clinical experience with strontium-89 in prostatic and breast cancer patients. Semin Oncol. 1993;20(3 Suppl 2):44-8.
67. **Janjan NA.** Radiation for bone metastases: conventional techniques and the role of systemic radiopharmaceuticals. Cancer. 1997;80(8 Suppl):1628-45.
68. **McEwan AJ.** Unsealed source therapy of painful bone metastases: an update. Semin Nucl Med. 1997;27:165-82.
69. **Coleman RE.** Management of bone metastases. ASCO Education Book, Spring 1998. Philadelphia: WB Saunders; 1998:100-8.
70. **Lewington VJ, McEwan AJ, Ackery DM, et al.** A prospective, randomised double-blind crossover study to examine the efficacy of strontium-89 in pain palliation in patients with advanced prostate cancer metastatic to bone. Eur J Cancer. 1991;27:954-8.
71. **Serafini AN, Houston SJ, Resche I, et al.** Palliation of pain associated with metastatic bone cancer using samarium-153 lexidronam: a double-blind placebo-controlled trial. J Clin Oncol. 1998;16:1574-81.
72. **Wycross RG.** Clinical experience with diamorphine in advanced malignant disease. Int J Clin Pharmacol. 1974;7:184-98.
73. **Kanner RM, Foley KM.** Patterns of narcotic drug use in a cancer pain clinic. Ann N Y Acad Sci. 1981;362:161-72.
74. **Porter J, Jick H.** Addiction rare in patients treated with narcotics [Letter]. N Engl J Med. 1980;302:123.
75. **Mercadante S.** Diarrhea, malabsorption, and constipation. In: Berger AM, Portenoy RK, Weissman DE, Eds. Principles and Practice of Supportive Oncology. Philadelphia: Lippincott-Raven; 1998:191-205.

76. Red Book. Montvale, NJ: Medical Economics; 1998.
77. **Vainio A, Ollila J, Matikainen E, et al.** Driving ability in cancer patients receiving long-term morphine analgesia. Lancet. 1995;346:667-70.
78. **Bruera E, Belzile M, Pituskin E, et al.** Randomized, double-blind, crossover trial comparing safety and efficacy of oral controlled-release oxycodone with controlled-release morphine in patients with cancer pain. J Clin Oncol. 1998;16:3222-9.
79. **Baines M.** Nausea and vomiting in the patient with advanced cancer. J Pain Symptom Manage. 1988;3:815.
80. **Currow DC, Coughlan M, Fardell B, Cooney NJ.** Use of ondansetron in palliative medicine. J Pain Symptom Manage. 1997;13:302-7.
81. **Ripamonti C.** Bowel obstruction. In: Berger AM, Portenoy RK, Weissman DE, Eds. Principles and Practice of Supportive Oncology. Philadelphia: Lippincott-Raven; 1998:207-16.
82. **Bruera E, Lawlor P, Watanabe S, et al.** The effects of opioid rotation (OR), dose ratio (DR) on pain control and cognition in patients (P) with cancer pain [Abstract]. Proc Am Soc Clin Oncol. 1997;16:62a.
83. **Lichter I.** Nausea and vomiting in patients with cancer. Hematol Oncol Clin North Am. 1996;10:207-20.
84. **Ripamonti C, Groff L, Brunelli C, et al.** Switching from morphine to oral methadone in treating cancer pain: what is the equianalgesic dose ratio? J Clin Oncol. 1998;16:3216-21.
85. **Mercadante S, Casuccio A, Agnello A, et al.** Morphine versus methadone in the pain treatment of advanced-cancer patients followed up at home. J Clin Oncol. 1998;16:3655-61.
86. **Foley KM, Houde RW.** Methadone in cancer pain management: individualize dose and titrate to effect [Editorial]. J Clin Oncol. 1998;16:3213-5.
87. **Manfredi PL, Ribeiro S, Chandler SW, Payne R.** Inappropriate use of naloxone in cancer patients with pain. J Pain Symptom Manage. 1996;11:131-4.
88. **Payne R.** Pharmacologic management of pain. In: Berger AM, Portenoy RK, Weissman DE, Eds. Principles and Practice of Supportive Oncology. Philadelphia: Lippincott-Raven; 1998:61-75.
89. **Caracini A, Martini C.** Neurological problems. In: Doyle D, Hanks GW, MacDonald N, Eds. Oxford Textbook of Palliative Medicine. 2nd ed. Oxford: Oxford University Press; 1997:727-49.
90. **Rodichok LD, Harper GR, Ruckdeschel JC, et al.** Early diagnosis of spinal epidural metastases. Am J Med. 1981;70:1181-8.
91. **Rodichok LD, Ruckdeschel JD, Harper GR, et al.** Early detection and treatment of spinal epidural metastases: the role of myelography. Ann Neurol. 1986;20:696-702.
92. **Portenoy RK, Galer BS, Salamon O, et al.** Identification of epidural neoplasm: radiography and bone scintigraphy in the symptomatic and asymptomatic spine. Cancer. 1989;64:2207-13.

93. **Portenoy RK, Lipton RB, Foley KM.** Back pain in the cancer patient: An algorithm for evaluation and management. Neurology. 1987;37:134-8.
94. **Hoskin PJ.** Radiotherapy in symptom management. In: Doyle D, Hanks GW, MacDonald N, Eds. Oxford Textbook of Palliative Medicine. 2nd ed. Oxford: Oxford University Press; 1997:267-82.
95. **Pinover WH, Coia LR.** Palliative radiation therapy. In: Berger AM, Portenoy RK, Weissman DE, Eds. Principles and Practice of Supportive Oncology. Philadelphia: Lippincott-Raven; 1998:603-26.
96. **Maranzano E, Latini P.** Effectiveness of radiation therapy without surgery in metastatic spinal cord compression: final results from a prospective trial. Int J Radiat Oncol Biol Phys. 1995;32:959-67.
97. **Siegal T, Siegal T.** Current considerations in the management of neoplastic spinal cord compression. Spine. 1989;14:223-8.
98. **Sorensen S, Helweg-Larsen S, Mouridsen H, Hansen HH.** Effect of high-dose dexamethasone in carcinomatous metastatic spinal cord compression treated with radiotherapy: a randomised trial. Eur J Cancer. 1994;30A:22-7.
99. **Heimdal K, Hirschberg H, Slettebo H, et al.** High incidence of serious side effects of high-dose dexamethasone treatment in patients with epidural spinal cord compression. J Neurooncol. 1992;12:141-4.
100. **Cobb CA III, Leavens ME, Eckles N.** Indications for nonoperative treatment of spinal cord compression due to breast cancer. J Neurosurg. 1977;47:653-8.
101. **Posner JB.** Neurological Complications of Cancer. Contemporary Neurology Series, vol 5. Philadelphia: FA Davis; 1995.
102. **Young RF, Post EM, King GA.** Treatment of spinal epidural metastases: randomized prospective comparison of laminectomy and radiotherapy. J Neurosurg. 1980;53:741-8.
103. **Findlay GF.** Adverse effects of the management of malignant spinal cord compression. J Neurol Neurosurg Psychiatry. 1984;47:761-8.
104. **Breitbart W, Chochinov HM, Passick S.** Psychiatric aspects of palliative care. In: Doyle D, Hanks GW, MacDonald N, Eds. Oxford Textbook of Palliative Medicine. 2nd ed. Oxford: Oxford University Press; 1997:933-54.
105. **Wilwerding MB, Loprinzi CL, Maillaird JA, et al.** A randomized, crossover evaluation of methylphenidate in cancer patients receiving strong narcotics. Support Care Cancer. 1995;3:135-8.
106. **Kreeger L, Duncan A, Cowap J.** Psychostimulants used for opioid-induced drowsiness [Letter]. J Pain Symptom Manage. 1996;11:1-2.
107. **Dalal S, Melzack R.** Potentiation of opioid analgesia by psychostimulant drugs: a review. J Pain Symptom Manage. 1998;16:245-53.
108. **Holland JC, ed.** Psycho-Oncology. New York: Oxford University Press; 1998.
109. **Saunders CM, Baines M.** Living with Dying: The Management of Terminal Disease. Oxford: Oxford University Press; 1989.
110. **Doyle D, Hanks GW, MacDonald N, Eds.** Oxford Textbook of Palliative Medicine. 2nd ed. Oxford: Oxford University Press; 1997.

111. **Berger AM, Portenoy RK, Weissman DE, Eds.** Principles and Practice of Supportive Oncology. Philadelphia: Lippincott-Raven; 1998:191-205.
112. **Waller A, Caroline NL.** Handbook of Palliative Care in Cancer. Boston: Butterworth-Heinemann; 1996.
113. **Storey P, Knight CF, Eds.** Hospice/Palliative Care Training for Physicians: A Self Study Program. 2nd ed. Reston, VA: American Academy of Hospice and Palliative Medicine; 1997.
114. **MacDonald N, Ed.** Palliative Medicine: A Case-Based Manual. Oxford: Oxford University Press; 1997.
115. Caring for the Dying: Identification and Promotion of Physician Competency. Philadelphia: American Board of Internal Medicine; 1996.

CHAPTER 6

Assessing and Managing Depression in the Terminally Ill Patient

SUSAN D. BLOCK, MD

Physicians who care for terminally ill patients commonly confront a range of complex medical and psychosocial challenges; treating patients who are experiencing psychosocial distress is often a particularly troublesome clinical task. Although it is difficult to imagine any patient facing the end of life without emotional distress, physicians may find it difficult to differentiate "normal," appropriate, and inevitable distress from more severe disturbances. In this chapter, we will use three cases to illustrate assessment and management of normal distress and grieving, clinical depression, and the wish to hasten death in the presence of psychological distress.

Why Should Physicians Treat Psychological Distress in the Terminally Ill?

Psychological distress impairs the patient's capacity for pleasure, meaning, and connection; erodes quality of life; amplifies pain and other symptoms (1-3); reduces the patient's ability to do the emotional work of separating and saying good-bye; and causes anguish and worry in family members and friends. Finally, psychological distress, particularly depression, is a major risk factor for suicide and for requests to hasten death (4).

What Are the Barriers to the Recognition and Treatment of Psychological Distress in the Terminally Ill?

Despite the well-documented prominence (5) of psychological distress in the dying, these problems tend to be underrecognized and undertreated (6). Numerous barriers exist to recognition and treatment of psychological symptoms in the terminally ill. Both patients and clinicians frequently believe that psychological distress is a normal feature of the dying process and fail to differentiate natural, existential distress from clinical depression. Physicians may lack the clinical knowledge and skills to identify problems such as depression, anxiety, and delirium, especially in the challenging clinical context of terminal illness when many of the usual diagnostic clues are confounded by co-existing medical illness and appropriate sadness (7). Many patients and physicians are reluctant to consider psychiatric etiologies for distress because of the stigma associated with such diagnoses, and both patients and clinicians often avoid exploration of psychological issues because of time constraints and concerns that they will cause further distress (8,9). Because physicians are reluctant to use psychotropics because of concern about additional adverse effects, many are hesitant to diagnose a condition that they are unconfident about effectively treating. Indeed, antidepressants account for only 1% to 5% of all psychotropics prescribed to cancer patients (10,11). Finally, physicians may feel a sense of hopelessness in caring for dying patients, which may lead to therapeutic nihilism (12).

How Prevalent is Psychological Distress in the Terminally Ill?

Psychological distress is a major cause of suffering among terminally ill patients and is highly correlated with poor quality of life (13). Indeed, more than 60% of cancer patients report experiencing distress. Differentiating the distress associated with the normal grieving that occurs as a person dies from the distress associated with psychiatric disorders requires an appreciation of the clinical characteristics and prevalence of these entities.

Derogatis et al found that 47% of cancer patients in varying stages of illness fulfilled the diagnostic criteria for psychiatric disorders (14). Sixty-eight percent of those with psychiatric disorders had adjustment disorders with depressed or anxious mood, 13% had major depression, and 8% had organic mental disorders (delirium). Information about the prevalence of psychiatric disorders in patients with other terminal illnesses demonstrates elevated rates relative to healthy populations (15).

CASE 6-1. SADNESS, GRIEF, OR DEPRESSION?

Mr. Roberts is a 53-year-old man with end-stage lung disease, cared for at home by his wife and the local hospice program. He receives chronic oxygen therapy, is bedbound, and has been hospitalized twice in the past year for respiratory failure requiring ventilatory support. Mr. Roberts is concerned about becoming a long-term burden to his children and wife. The family's income is barely enough to meet their needs. Recently, the hospice nurse has expressed concern about Mr. Roberts' mental state because he has been asking repeatedly why he has to wait around to die. When directly questioned, he states that he has no intention of ending his life but is distressed by his helplessness and dependence. He says he feels like "a time-bomb ticking." He spends his time watching television and trying to complete two woodworking projects.

The physician hearing this report must assess the severity and possible interventions for Mr. Roberts' distress. Is he depressed, or is he experiencing the normal grieving that is part of the dying process? What is the appropriate threshold for diagnosing depression? In addition, the physician confronts the challenge of contending with the patient's distress while remaining present as a witness and an ally in traversing this difficult passage. The clinical features of grief and depression are contrasted in Table 6-1.

Our knowledge of psychological disorders in terminally ill patients comes predominantly from patients with AIDS and cancer and from

Table 6-1. Grief Versus Depression in Terminal Illness.

Grief	Depression
Feeling or emotion and behaviors resulting from a particular loss (16).	Constellation of feelings, emotions, and behaviors that fulfill criteria for major psychiatric disorder; distress is usually generalized to all facets of life.
Universal; only a minority of grieving patients develop full-blown affective disorders requiring treatment.	Prevalence of major depression is 1%-53% (17-22).
Patients usually cope with distress on their own.	Medical/psychiatric intervention usually necessary.
Somatic distress; loss of usual patterns of behavior; agitation, sleep, and appetite disturbances; decreased concentration; social withdrawal.	Similar symptoms, plus hopelessness, helplessness, worthlessness, guilt, and suicidal ideation (23-27).
Associated with disease progression.	Increased prevalence (up to 77%) with advanced disease (28); pain is a major risk factor (29-31).
Patient retains capacity for pleasure.	Nothing is enjoyable.
Comes in waves.	Constant, unremitting.
Passive wishes for death to come quickly.	Intense and persistent suicidal ideation.
Able to look forward to the future.	No sense of positive future.

geriatric patients. There is relatively little published literature about psychological issues affecting patients with end-stage pulmonary, cardiac, renal, and neurologic disease. Thus, the recommendations in this paper about the treatment of distressed patients at the end of life represent extrapolations from existing literature and expert opinion but lack specific evidence of efficacy in some populations.

How is Depression Diagnosed in the Terminally Ill?

The physician makes a house call to further assess Mr. Roberts' condition. Throughout the visit, Mr. Roberts makes cheerful jokes about his condition ("Hey, Doc, I'm not dead yet") and refers repeatedly to his death in a joking manner. The physician elicits information that Mr. Roberts is not sleeping well because he is short of breath and is anxious about falling asleep and not waking up, that his appetite is poor, and that he has little energy. He reports that he doesn't want to see anyone outside of his family, and that he lacks the concentration and focus to read. When asked whether he is depressed, Mr. Roberts replies, "Depressed? That word holds no meaning for me. Angry, yes. Fed up, yes. Worried about my family, yes. But depression? Never." He remarks on how much he enjoys his woodworking projects and worries that he won't have time to complete them. He speaks about his pleasure in visiting with his sons. Then, he says, "This dying thing can't be over quick enough or last long enough for me." Mr. Roberts reports that he is realistic about his prognosis, hopes for a few more good months, is trying to do as much as possible for himself, and is not suicidal. He says joking has always been his way of coping with difficult situations.

Mr. Roberts presents many of the common challenges in diagnosing depression (32). He has several of the neurovegetative symptoms of depression (difficulty sleeping, poor appetite, loss of energy, diminished concentration). However, these symptoms may be caused or exacerbated by his underlying pulmonary disease. Mr. Roberts also is grieving as he anticipates his death. His withdrawal from people outside his family is likely to be part of the normal grieving process, particularly because he continues to enjoy his visits with his children. Like others, the patient expresses ambivalence about the prospect of death, simultaneously accepting and denying it (33).

The clinical interview is the "gold standard" for the diagnosis of depression (34,35). Chochinov et al found that the single question "Are you depressed?" provides a sensitive and specific assessment of depression in the terminally ill (36). A patient who responds affirmatively to such an inquiry has a high likelihood of receiving a diagnosis of depression after a comprehensive diagnostic interview. The busy physician can use this question to screen patients for depression. Mr. Roberts' response that he is not depressed is important evidence weighing against the diagnosis of depression. Table 6-2 summarizes the indicators of depression that are most useful in the diagnosis of patients with terminal illness.

Table 6-2.   Clues to the Diagnosis of Depression in the Terminally Ill.

Psychological Symptoms
  Dysphoria
  Depressed mood
  Sadness
  Tearfulness
  Lack of pleasure
  Hopelessness
  Helplessness
  Worthlessness
  Social withdrawal
  Guilt
  Suicidal ideation
Other Indicators
  Intractable pain or other symptoms
  Excessive somatic preoccupation
  Disproportionate disability
  Poor cooperation or treatment refusal (37)
  Hopelessness, aversion, lack of interest on the part of the clinician (38,39)
  Treatment with corticosteroids, interferon, etc.
History
  Personal or family history of substance abuse, depression or bipolar illness
  Pancreatic cancer (40)

In assessing these psychological symptoms, physicians must contextualize the patient's responses. For example, the patient's illness may be grounds for realistic hopelessness: the patient may, in fact, be quite helpless because of his or her physical condition; role loss because of illness may result in loss of self-esteem; and a patient whose illness is related to behavioral patterns (e.g., smoking) may feel a sense of guilt for causing the illness. Nevertheless, when these symptoms are out of proportion to the patient's actual situation, they are useful indicators of the presence of a major depression. The physician can also attend to his or her own emotional responses to the patient as a diagnostic clue. Patients with depression often engender feelings of boredom, hopelessness, aversion, and lack of interest in their caregivers, mirroring the dysphoria, hopelessness, and self-criticism that are hallmarks of the patient's experience of depression (41). The physician noted that he enjoyed Mr. Roberts' mordant sense of humor and was amused by his delight in shocking the hospice nurse with his jokes, further evidence that Mr. Roberts is not depressed.

Because Mr. Roberts' distress is focused around real issues related to his illness (the burden of care on his family, uncertainty, distress about loss of control), and because he retains the capacity to laugh, to be involved in his hobbies, and to enjoy his family, the physician concludes that Mr. Roberts is not depressed and that his distress appears to fall within the rubric of what the DSM-IV calls "adjustment disorders" (42). The physician suggests that the hospice nurse continue to monitor his mood and recommends a trial of an antidepressant only if he demonstrates new depressive symptoms.

Because there is no "bright line" between depression and grief or adjustment reactions, the physician must assess whether the patient's symptoms have reached the threshold for treatment. Psychological distress, even when it does not reach the threshold of a psychiatric diagnosis, requires treatment. Many of the treatments (listening, exploration of concerns, reinforcement of the patient's coping strengths, facilitation of dialogue with family members) are part of the clinician's responsibility. The interventions that involve the physician as a healing agent (43) can result in marked improvements in the patient's adaptation. In general, because the available drug treatments for depression have become easier to use and tend to have fewer side effects than older medications, a strong case can also be made for a therapeutic trial of antidepressant medication when the diagnosis is in question. Treatment with psychostimulants (see below) can provide a relatively quick test of whether antidepressants are likely to be effective.

Although he frequently expressed worry about the impact of his illness on his family, Mr. Roberts continued to cope with his illness and his approaching death with black humor. He died peacefully at home 3 months later.

CASE 6-2. ASSESSMENT AND MANAGEMENT OF DEPRESSION

Ms. Ferrone is a 78-year-old woman with metastatic breast cancer with bone and liver metastases who is receiving palliative chemotherapy. She is Roman Catholic and lives with her husband and 40-year-old retarded daughter. In the past 6 months, she has fractured two vertebrae and been hospitalized for a pulmonary embolus. She and her family have always wanted aggressive treatment, primarily so that she could con-

tinue to care for her daughter. Recently, however, she has said that she is too sick to be of help to anyone and that she does not want further treatment. She has pain that is poorly controlled with pamidronate, naproxen, and morphine. Her current pain levels are at best a 3 and at worst a 7 on a 10-point scale. She notes that pain often interferes with her sleep and that she cannot sleep past 4 a.m. Her appetite is poor, and she has lost interest in her hobbies.

Because of the change in her status, the physician carries out a depression assessment. When asked about her future, Ms. Ferrone responds, "My future is over. There is nothing good ahead for me. I worry about how much suffering is ahead, about my daughter, and about how my husband will manage. If it weren't for my religion, I would call that doctor who kills people. I used to feel proud of being a good mother and wife. But I've lost that. All I can see is how much suffering I am putting people through. I can't forgive myself for that." When asked whether she thinks she is depressed, Ms. Ferrone says that she is nervous and sad, and that she feels that anyone would be depressed in her circumstances.

This case presents a number of indicators that Ms. Ferrone suffers from clinical depression. Physicians caring for terminally ill patients should consider the diagnosis of depression when a patient unexpectedly elects to discontinue treatment, is experiencing unrelieved pain, or demonstrates any of the neurovegetative symptoms of depression. In addition, particularly with geriatric patients, the diagnosis of depression should be entertained for patients who complain about memory problems or who demonstrate elevated levels of somatic concern. A clinician can fully evaluate depressive symptoms in this clinical context by asking questions such as:

- How do you see your future?
- What do you imagine is ahead for yourself with this illness?
- What aspects of your life do you feel most proud of? Most troubled by?
- Are you depressed?

Ms. Ferrone's response to her physician's questions suggests that she is feeling hopeless and depressed. She is unable to imagine anything positive in her future, feels unable to contribute, and believes that her presence is only a burden to others. Although her religious beliefs make suicide unlikely, clearly she has some wish to end her life. Many patients and clinicians believe that depression is a normal feature of terminal illness; however, most patients do not become depressed in the setting of terminal illness (44). Feelings of hopelessness, helplessness, worthlessness, guilt, and suicidal ideation, all present in Ms. Ferrone, are among the best indicators of depression in terminally ill patients. Anxiety commonly coexists with depression, and some patients experience an anxious depression (45,46). In addition, organic mental disorders (e.g., delirium) caused by metastatic disease or paraneoplastic syndromes may mimic depression (47). A medical evaluation should be completed to assess possible organic contributors to depressed mood. Components of the appropriate medical evaluation will vary depending on the patient's clinical situation.

How Should Depression Be Treated in a Terminally Ill Patient?

The first step in assessing and treating depression is controlling pain. Uncontrolled pain is a major risk factor for both depression and suicide among cancer patients (48,49). Sixty to ninety percent of cancer patients experience pain during the last year of life (50-52); more than 90% of patients with cancer pain respond to simple analgesic measures (53,54). The SUPPORT study demonstrated that even hospitalized patients with diseases not usually considered to be painful (e.g., cardiac disease) were reported by their families to experience moderate to severe pain (55).

Ms. Ferrone's analgesics were increased and her pain control improved. Although her mood brightened slightly, she continued to express hopelessness about the future and showed no improvement in her other mood symptoms.

Major depression is a highly treatable condition, even among the terminally ill. Because treatments are usually relatively benign, experts recommend that clinicians have a low threshold for initiating treatment.

Trials of individual interventions demonstrate the effectiveness of psychotherapeutic interventions in relieving distress (56,57), improving quality of life (58-60), and even in prolonging life (61), and the effectiveness of psychopharmacologic interventions in relieving depressive symptoms and psychological distress in as many as 80% of patients (62). Although there are no controlled clinical trials to evaluate the efficacy of combined interventions, most experts recommend an approach that combines supportive psychotherapy, patient and family education, and antidepressants (63). Unfortunately, few of the reported trials, including those of psychopharmacologic agents, meet the most rigorous standards for evidence-based practice, and most of the research has been carried out with cancer patients. Additionally, few of these interventions have been systematically evaluated with terminally ill patients.

Psychotherapy and Counseling

In developing a treatment strategy, it is essential that the clinician elicit the patient's concerns through active questioning about fears of death and the dying process, concerns about the impact of illness on family members, and past experiences with loss. By addressing these concerns, the physician can help the patient connect with past strengths and assets, spiritual and religious resources, self-esteem enhancement, and coping ability. Sometimes, supportive therapy alone is sufficient to treat depression. Supportive therapy can be delivered by a psychiatrist, psychologist, social worker, hospice nurse, or primary care physician, depending on time, interest, and training, and on the severity of the patient's condition. Terminally ill patients benefit from an approach that combines emotional support, flexibility, appreciation of the patient's strengths, and elements of life review to assist the patient in coming to a sense of closure and completion of her/his life. The physician's ability to convey a vision of the potential for connection, meaning, reconciliation, and closure in the dying process is thought to facilitate the patient's ability to come to terms with impending death (64). However, patients with severe depressive symptoms may be too immobilized, hopeless, and dysphoric to engage effectively in psychotherapy until they have received appropriate antidepressant medication.

Psychopharmacology

Psychostimulants, selective serotonin reuptake inhibitors (SSRIs), and tricyclic antidepressants (TCAs) are the mainstay of treatment for depressed, terminally ill patients (65). They are particularly useful for patients who are seriously ill and may be unable to engage in psychotherapy (66). Characteristics of these agents are described in Table 6-3. Although a variety of new antidepressants have been introduced in recent years, these drugs have not yet been evaluated for use in terminally ill patients.

Psychostimulants (dextroamphetamine, methylphenidate, and pemoline) deserve special consideration in treating depression near the end of life. For patients with a limited lifespan, a rapid onset of action reduces patient and family distress and creates opportunities for the patient and family to cope more effectively with the challenges of the dying process. Even patients who are quite debilitated and fatigued may experience an improvement in mood and energy within 24 hours of starting treatment.

However, psychostimulants are not the drugs of choice for terminally ill patients who have relatively long projected lifespans; they are best used in patients with weeks to several months to live. For patients with severe depression who require urgent treatment but who are anticipated to survive for several months or longer, it is often useful to initiate treatment with a psychostimulant, adding an SSRI (see below) after the patient has a therapeutic response to the psychostimulant, and titrating the patient off the psychostimulant and onto the SSRI during 1-2 weeks.

Despite their efficacy and relative lack of side effects, many physicians are reluctant to prescribe psychostimulants because of concerns about side effects and liability through the Controlled Substances Act. These agents are, however, well-accepted treatments in the psychiatric literature for depressed medically ill patients.

The SSRIs (fluoxetine, paroxetine, and sertraline) are often the first-line agents for treatment of depression in the terminally ill when immediate onset of action is not essential. In general, paroxetine or sertraline are better tolerated by terminally ill patients because they have fewer active metabolites that can accumulate and cause toxicity.

Although tricyclic antidepressants are still used in terminally ill patients, their sedating and autonomic effects make them less well-tolerated than the SSRIs. Because of the proliferation of new antidepressants, including many not mentioned here, the internist is best served by becoming familiar with the risks and benefits of a small subset of available antidepressants in each class, using them when clinically indicated, and referring patients who do not improve on these agents for psychiatric consultation.

Table 6-3. Antidepressants for Use in Terminally Ill Patients.

Class of Agent	Quality of Evidence	Advantages	Disadvantages	Onset of Action	Starting Dose (mg)	Usual Daily Dose (mg)	Maximal Daily Dose (mg)	Side Effects	Schedule
Psychostimulants	Anecdotal reports, retrospective case reviews, small controlled prospective trials (67,68)	Rapid onset of action; well tolerated in elderly and debilitated patients; effective adjuvant analgesics (69,70); counter opioid-induced fatigue; improve appetite (71) and energy; effectiveness 70% (72) to 82% (73); useful in treating cognitive impairment in AIDS (74)	Cardiac decompensation can occur in elderly patients, and patients with heart disease; confusion in old or cognitively impaired patients (75); tolerance may develop but occurs infrequently		Start low, titrate upwards q1–2 days until therapeutic response, side effects, or maximal dose reached			Mean side effects = 11%: restlessness, dizziness, nightmares, insomnia, palpitations, arrhythmia, tremor, dry mouth; psychosis rare; pemoline produces minimal cardiac stimulation	
Methylphenidate				<24 hr	2.5–5	10–20	60–90		8 A.M. & Noon
Dextroamphetamine				<24 hr	2.5	5–10	60–90		Once daily
Pemoline			Hepatocellular injury and choreoathetosis; hepatic function must be monitored regularly; use with caution in patients with renal failure	1–2 days	18.75	37.5	150		Once daily

Drug	Efficacy	Comments	Interactions	Time to response	Starting dose (mg)	Therapeutic dose (mg)	Maximum dose (mg)	Adverse effects	Schedule
SSRIs	Controlled, double-blind studies demonstrate superiority over placebo in depression (76), HIV-related depression (77), and depression with heart disease (78); SSRIs are as safe and effective as TCAs for depression (79,80); no controlled studies in terminal illness	Safe and effective with few side effects; little orthostatic hypotension, urinary retention, sedation; no effects on cardiac conduction; easy to titrate	Inhibt P4502D6 causing interactions with other drugs; fluoxetine has long half-life	2–4 wk				Paroxetine and sertraline better tolerated than fluoxetine (81); nausea, GI distress, insomnia, headache, sexual dysfunction, anorexia	Once daily
Sertraline					12.5–25	50–100	200		
Fluoxetine					5–10	20–40	60		
Paroxetine					10	20–40	60		
Tricyclics	Multiple studies demonstrate efficacy in depressed medically ill patients (82), but none are controlled	Therapeutic response often seen at low dose; effective for treatment of neuropathic pain (83); can be given parenterally or compounded for rectal administration; drug levels can be monitored (84)	Nortriptyline and desipramine better tolerated than amitryptiline and imipramine (85); amitryptyline and doxepin can be used as sleep medications	2–4 wk				Adverse effects occur in as many as 34% of cancer patients (62); not well tolerated in terminally ill patients due to anticholinergic side effects (dry mouth, delirium, constipation, etc.)	Qhs
Amitryptyline					10–25	25–100	150		
Imipramine					10–25	25–100	150		
Doxepin					10–25	25–100	150		
Desipramine					10–25	25–100	150		
Nortriptyline					10–25	25–75	125		

Although Ms. Ferrone was reluctant to start medication because she felt that she should be "glad to go to God," she agreed to start on methylphenidate 2.5 mg po at 8 a.m. and noon. Within two days, her family noted that that she had more energy, was sleeping better, and reported less pain. Her methylphenidate was increased; several days later, she reported that she was feeling less downhearted and that even though she didn't want any more aggressive treatment she was looking forward to the holidays. Within 10 days, Ms. Ferrone's family felt that she was back to her previous baseline. She entered a hospice program and was maintained on methylphenidate without recurrence of her depression. After her death, Ms. Ferrone's family expressed their gratitude that "she had remained herself until the very end."

In understanding and treating depression, the clinician must recognize that the meanings and expression of depressive symptoms may vary across cultures (85). Some patients who have strong beliefs in an afterlife may struggle to reconcile views of death as an opportunity to be closer to God, whereas others may fear hell and damnation. These varying perceptions influence the patient's response to terminal illness. Furthermore, some cultures stigmatize psychiatric disorders, and both patients and their families may be reluctant to acknowledge depressive symptoms and to accept treatment. Often, the additional expertise of respected leaders from the patient's own culture or religious orientation can be helpful in encouraging a patient to accept treatment.

CASE 6-3. ASSESSMENT AND MANAGEMENT OF SUICIDAL IDEATION IN THE TERMINALLY ILL

Mr. Wyznyski is a 36-year-old man with AIDS who recently stopped his antiretroviral treatment because of side effects. He lives with his partner near his family. Mr. Wyznyski recently stopped work because he was too ill but has remained active in AIDS education programs. Ten years ago, he nursed his former partner as he died from AIDS. Mr. Wyznyski has been open with his partner, family, and physician about his inten-

tion to end his life if his suffering becomes unbearable. He has a severe peanut allergy and intends to consume a nut-filled candy bar if he becomes intolerably ill. During the past several months, Mr. Wyznyski has become blind because of cytomegalovirus retinitis and is wheelchair-bound because of peripheral neuropathy. His Kaposi's sarcoma has proliferated, and he has lost 35 pounds. Nonetheless, he has continued to be active in his teaching activities. He comes to his regularly scheduled visit saying that he has come to say good-bye and thank you for the care he has received, and that he plans to kill himself within a few days. Although Mr. Wyznyski has been considering suicide as a theoretical option, he now appears to have an immediate plan.

Assessment of the patient's suicide risk will be informed by an appreciation of the fact that the rates of suicide in patients with medical illness are elevated and rise as illness progresses (86). Additional risk factors for suicide in terminally ill patients include advanced age, male gender, diagnoses of cancer or AIDS, depression, hopelessness, delirium, exhaustion, pain, pre-existing psychopathology, and personal or family history of suicide (87-89). Suicidal thoughts occur in as many as 45% of terminally ill cancer patients and are usually fleeting and associated with feelings of loss of control and anxiety about the future. However, in a study of a small number of terminally ill cancer patients, 8.5% of terminally ill cancer patients expressed a sustained and pervasive wish for death to come quickly, and 59% of these patients were diagnosed as depressed (4). These patients were found to have elevated levels of pain and low social supports. It is not known whether treatment of depression results in diminished desire for early death, but in a study of depressed geriatric patients' preferences for life-sustaining therapy Ganzini et al found that more than 25% of severely depressed patients who initially refused treatment showed increased desire for life-sustaining treatment after improvement of depressive symptoms (90).

Table 6-4 outlines an approach to the assessment of suicidality. Even patients who present the desire for suicide as a "rational" choice should receive a comprehensive assessment. The approach to patients who desire hastened death has been reviewed elsewhere (91,92).

Table 6-4. Assessing Suicidality in the Terminally Ill Patient.

1. Examine patient's reasons for wanting to end his/her life now
   Explore the meanings of patient's desire to die
2. Assess pain and symptom control
   Is untreated or undertreated pain contributing to the desire to die?
   Are untreated or undertreated other symptoms contributing to the desire to die?
   Are fears about the dying process contributing to the desire to die?
   Is the patient experiencing medication side effects that can be ameliorated?
3. Review patient's social supports
   Has there been a recent loss, conflict, or rejection?
   Are there new fears of abandonment or rejection?
   With whom has patient spoken about his/her plan?
   How do they feel about the patient's plan?
4. Assess cognitive status
   Are there cognitive deficits?
   Are there new neurologic signs or symptoms?
   Does patient understand his/her condition, its implications, and the implications of suicide?
   Is the patient's judgment distorted by hopelessness and other symptoms of depression?
5. Assess psychological condition
   Does the patient have untreated or undertreated anxiety, depression, panic disorder, delirium, or other psychiatric diagnosis?
   How is the patient dealing with issues of loss of control, dependency, uncertainty, grief?
6. Explore religious, spiritual, and existential concerns
   Are there unresolved or distressing questions or concerns in these domains?

Involving Other Health Professionals in Assessment and Treatment

In carrying out this assessment, the physician must remain involved and rely on the expertise of other members of an interdisciplinary team. Several circumstances should prompt a referral to a psychiatrist (Table 6-5). Psychiatrists with expertise in the assessment and management of patients with severe medical illness can be found in most major medical centers as part of medical psychiatry or consultation-liaison psychiatry services. A psychiatrist can provide an in-depth assessment of the patient's judgment, decision-making capacity, and mood.

Table 6-5. Circumstances That Should Prompt Psychiatric Referral.

- Uncertainty about psychiatric diagnosis
- Past history of major psychiatric disorder
- Patient suicidal
- Patient requesting assisted suicide/euthanasia
- Patient psychotic/confused
- Patient unresponsive to first-line antidepressants
- Dysfunctional family dynamics

A social worker can provide critical information about the patient's social network and coping. A chaplain can provide insight about the patient's spiritual concerns.

Although some clinicians are concerned that exploration of suicidal thoughts may exacerbate the thoughts, there is no evidence that this occurs. The current standard of practice suggests that patients who show pervasive hopelessness or persistent desire to die should be referred to a psychiatrist for assessment and treatment because of their high risk for suicide (93). The presence of hallucinations or delusions in depressed patients should be viewed as indicators of high risk for suicide (94). Similarly, organic mental disorders, especially among AIDS patients, are also risk factors (95). Although psychiatric hospitalization is rarely indicated in this circumstance for terminally ill patients, mobilization of supports, attention to sources of suffering and meaning, affirmation of the person's value, and treatment with antidepressants and/or antipsychotics are often successful in helping the patient want to carry on.

> *The physician explores Mr. Wyznyski's decision to end his life now and asks the social worker and chaplain for their input. Although Mr. Wyznyski is initially angry that the physician questions his intention to kill himself, his anger dissipates and he begins to cry when his physician says, "We've been through this whole rotten disease together. I am not going to abandon you now. We both know that your time is short, but I want to help you have the best possible death you can have." Mr. Wyznyski says that he is tired of fighting and trying to be a role model. He is afraid of letting people down by giving up. He says, "I never thought I would say this, but death has become*

my friend. I don't have the energy to get up and get dressed and try to put on a good face." With Mr. Wyznyski's agreement, the physician and social worker arrange a family meeting where these concerns are shared. Mr. Wyznyski's family and partner explain that they recognize how exhausted he has become but acknowledge that they have been afraid to encourage him to slow down because they don't want to demoralize him. After the meeting, Mr. Wyznyski says that he feels relieved that he doesn't have to work so hard to keep up appearances. He gives up his teaching engagements, spending his days in bed, and dies a month later.

Discussion

We have reviewed three cases illustrating the assessment and management of normal or appropriate grieving, the diagnosis and treatment of depression, and assessment and management of suicidal ideation among the terminally ill. Skillful management of depression relieves suffering in the patient and is a core element of the provision of comprehensive end-of-life care. Although treatment of pain and other symptoms at the end of life has improved, depression and other psychological symptoms remain among the most troublesome symptoms for patients facing the end of life. Many of these symptoms are readily controllable using state-of-the-art psychosocial treatments. All physicians who care for dying patients should be competent in this critical domain of clinical practice.

Acknowledgements

This work was supported by NIH Grant CA66818-05, the Project on Death in America, the Robert Wood Johnson Foundation, and the Nathan Cummings Foundation. I appreciate the secretarial support of Cheryl Adamick.

REFERENCES

1. **Massie MJ, Holland JC.** The cancer patient with pain: psychiatric complications and their management. Med Clin North Am. 1987;71:243-8.
2. **Dean C.** Psychiatric morbidity following mastectomy: preoperative predictors and types of illness. J Psychosom Res. 1987;31:385-92.

3. **Breitbart W, Bruera E, Chochinov H, Lynch M.** Neuropsychiatric syndromes and psychological symptoms in patients with advanced cancer. J Pain Symp Manage. 1995;10:131-41.

4. **Chochinov HM, Wilson KG, Enns M, et al.** Desire for death in the terminally ill. Am J Psychiatry. 1995;152:1185-91.

5. **Kaasa S, Malt U, Hagen S, et al.** Psychological distress in cancer patients with advanced disease. Radiother Oncol. 1993;27:193-7.

6. **Stiefel FC, Kornblith AB, Holland JC.** Changes in the prescription patterns of psychotropic drugs for cancer patients during a 10-year period. Cancer. 1990;65:1048-53.

7. **McCartney CF, et al.** Effect of psychiatric liaison program on consultation rates and on detection of minor psychiatric disorders in cancer patients. Am J Psychiatry. 1989;7:898-901.

8. **Comaroff J, Maguire P.** Ambiguity and the search for meaning: childhood leukemia in the modern clinical context. Soc Sci Med. 1981;15B:115-123.

9. **Maguire P.** The recognition and treatment of affective disorders in cancer patients. Int Rev Appl Psychol. 1984;33:479-91.

10. **Derogatis LR, Feldstein M, Morrow G, et al.** A survey of psychotropic drug prescriptions in an oncology population. Cancer. 1979;44:1919-29.

11. **Jaeger H, Morrow GT, Brescia F.** A survey of psychotropic drug utilizaiton by patients with advanced neoplastic disease. Gen Hosp Psychiatry. 1985;7:353-60.

12. **Block SD, Billings JA.** Patient requests to hasten death: evaluation and management in terminal care. Arch Intern Med. 1994;154:2039-47.

13. **Portenoy, RK, Thaler HT, Kornblith AB, et al.** Symptom prevalence, characteristics, and distress in a cancer population. Qual Life Res. 1994;3:183-9.

14. **Derogatis LR, Marrow GR, Fetting J, et al.** The prevalence of psychiatric disorders among cancer patients. JAMA. 1983;249:751-7.

15. **Cassem EH.** Depressive disorders in the medically ill: an overview. Psychosomatics. 1995;36:S2-S10.

16. **Osterweis, M, Solomon, F, Green M, Eds.** Bereavement: Reactions, Consequences, and Care. Washington, DC: National Academy Press; 1984.

17. **Breitbart W.** Suicide in cancer patients. Oncology. 1987;1:49-54.

18. **Weisman AD.** Coping behavior and suicide in cancer. In: Cullen JW, Fox BH, Isom RN, Eds. Cancer: The Behavioral Dimensions. New York: Raven Press; 1976.

19. **Bolund C.** Suicide and cancer: I. Demographic and social characteristics of cancer patients who committed suicide in Sweden, 1973-1976. J Psychosoc Oncol. 1985;3:17-30.

20. **Bolund C.** Suicide and cancer: II. Medical and care factors in suicides by cancer patients in Sweden, 1973-1976. J Psychosoc Oncol. 1985:3:31-52.

21. **Chochinov HM, Wilson KG, Enns M, Lander S.** Prevalence of depression in the terminally ill: effects of diagnostic criteria and symptom threshold judgment. Am J Psychiatry. 1994;151:537-40.

22. **DeFlorio M, Massie MJ.** Review of depression in cancer: gender differences. Depression. 1995;2:66-80.
23. **Plumb MM, Holland J.** Comparative studies of psychological function in patients with advanced cancer I. Self-reported depressive symptoms. Psychosom Med. 1977;39:264-76.
24. **Plumb MM, Holland JC.** Comparative studies of psychological function in patients with advanced cancer: II. Interviewer-rated current and past psychological symptoms. Psychosom Med. 1981;43:243-54.
25. **Lindemann E.** Symptomatology and management of acute grief. Am J Psychiatry 1944;101:141-8.
26. **Brown JT, Stoudemire GA.** Normal and pathological grief. JAMA. 1983;250:378-82.
27. **Clayton P.** Mourning and depression: their similarities and differences. Can J Psychiatry. 1974;1:309-12.
28. **Bukberg J, Penman D, Holland J.** Depression in hospitalized cancer patients. Psychosom Med. 1984;43:199-212.
29. **Ahles TA, Blanchard EB, Ruckdeschel JC.** The multidimensional nature of cancer-related pain. Pain. 1983;17:277-88.
30. **Woodforde JM, Fielding JR.** Pain and cancer. J Psychosom Res. 1970;14:365-70.
31. **Spiegel D, Sands S, Koopman C.** Pain and depression in patients with cancer. Cancer. 1994;74:2570-8.
32. **Kathol RG, Noyes R, Williams J, et al.** Diagnosing depression in patients with medical illness. Psychosomatics. 1990;31:434-40.
33. **Weisman A.** On Dying and Denying: a Psychiatric Study of Terminality. New York: Behavioral Publications; 1972.
34. **Koenig HG, Cohen JH, Blazer DG.** A brief depression scale for use in the medically ill. Int J Psychiatr Med. 1992;22:183-95.
35. **Gerety MG, Williams JW Jr., Mulrow CD, et al.** Performance of case-finding tools for depression in the nursing home: influence of clinical and functional characteristics and selection of optimal threshold scores. J Am Geriatr Soc. 1994;42:1103-9.
36. **Chochinov HM, Wilson KG, Enns M, Lander S.** "Are you depressed?" Screening for depression in the terminally ill. Am J Psychiatry. 1997;154:674-5.
37. **Goldberg RJ.** Systematic understanding of cancer patients who refuse treatment. Psychother Psychosom. 1983;39:1507-12.
38. **Maltsburger JT, Buie DH.** Countertransferance hate in the treatment of suicidal patients. Arch Gen Psych. 1974;30:625-33.
39. **Burt R.** Taking Care of Strangers. New York: Free Press; 1979.
40. **Holland JC, Hughes AH, Tross S, et al.** Comparative psychological disturbance in patients with pancreatic and gastric cancer. Am J Psychiatry. 1986;143:982-6.
41. **Groves J.** Taking care of the hateful patient. N Engl J Med. 1978;298:883-7.

42. **American Psychiatric Association.** Diagnostic and Statistical Manual of Mental Disorders. 4th ed. Washington, DC: American Psychiatric Association: 1994.

43. **Balint M.** The Doctor, His Patient, and the Illness. New York: International Universities Press; 1972.

44. **Breitbart W, Krivo S.** Suicide. In: Holland JC, Ed. Psychooncology. New York: Oxford University Press; 1998.

45. **Zinberg RE, Barlow DH.** Mixed anxiety-depression: a new diagostic category. In: Rapee RM, Barlow DH, Eds. Chronic Anxiety: Generalized Anxiety Disorder and Mixed Anxiety-Depression. New York: Guilford Press; 1991;136-52.

46. **Liebowitz MR.** Mixed anxiety and depression: should it be included in DSM-IV? J Clin Psychiatry. 1993;54(Suppl):4-7.

47. **Levine PM, Silberfarb PM, Lipowski ZJ.** Mental disorders in cancer patients. Cancer. 1978; 42:1385-91.

48. **Breitbart W.** Cancer pain and suicide. In: Foley KM, Bonica JJ, Ventafridda V, Eds. Advances in Pain Research and Therapy. New York: Raven Press; 1990.

49. **Helig S.** The San Francisco Medical Society euthanasia survey. Results and analysis. San Francisco Medicine. 1988;61:24-34.

50. **Twycross RG, Lack SA.** Symptom Control in Far Advanced Cancer: Pain Relief. London: Pitman Publishing; 1984.

51. **Cleeland CS.** The impact of pain on patients with cancer. Cancer. 1984;54:235-41.

52. **Portenoy RK.** Cancer pain: pathophysiology and syndromes. Lancet. 1992;339:1026-31.

53. **Ventafridda V, Tamburini M, Caraceni A, et al.** A validation study of the WHO method for cancer pain relief. Cancer. 1987;59:350-6.

54. **Grond S, Zech D, Schug SA, et al.** Validation of World Health Organization guidelines for cancer pain relief during the last days and hours of life. J Pain Symp Manage. 1991;6:411-22.

55. **SUPPORT Principal Investigators.** A controlled trial to improve care for seriously ill hospitalized patients. JAMA. 1995;274:1591-8.

56. **Greer S, Moorey S, Baruch JDR, et al.** Adjuvant psychological therapy for patients with cancer: a prospective randomised trial. BMJ. 1992;304:675-80.

57. **Spiegel D, Bloom JR, Yalom I.** Group support for patients with metastatic cancer: a randomized prospective outcome study. Arch Gen Psychiatry. 1981;38:527-33.

58. **Fallowfield LJ, Hall A, Maguire GP, et al.** Psychological outcomes of different treatment policies in women with early breast cancer outside a clinical trial. BMJ. 1990;301:575-80.

59. **Fawzy FI, Cousins N, Fawzy NW, et al.** A structured psychiatric intervention for cancer patients: I. Arch Gen Psychiatry. 1990;47:720-5.

60. **Fawzy FI, Kemeny ME, Fawzy NW, et al.** A structured psychiatric intervention for cancer patients: II. Arch Gen Psychiatry. 1990:47:729-35.

61. **Spiegel D, Kraemer HC, Bloom JR, Gottheil E.** Effect of psychosocial treatment on survival of patients with metastatic breast cancer. Lancet. 1989; 888-91.

62. **Chaturvedi, Maguire P, Hopwood P.** Antidepressant medications in cancer patients. Psycho-Oncology. 1994;3:57-60.

63. **Massie MJ, Holland JC.** Depression and the cancer patient. J Clin Psychiatry. 1990;51:12-17.

64. **Byock I.** Dying Well: The Prospect for Growth at the End of Life. New York: Riverhead Books; 1997.

65. **Katon W, Sullivan MD.** Depression and chronic medical illness. J Clin Psychiatry. 1990;51:6(Suppl):3-11.

66. **Maguire GP, Hopwood P, Tarrier N, et al.** Treatment of depression in cancer patients. Acta Psychiat Scand. 1985;72:81-4.

67. **Masand PS, Tesar GE.** Use of stimulants in the medically ill. Psychiatr Clin North Am. 1996;19:515-47.

68. **Fernandez F, Adams F, Holmes VF, et al.** Methylphenidate for depressive disorders in cancer patients: an alternative to standard antidepressants. Psychosomatics. 1987;28:455-62.

69. **Bruera R, Fainsinger R, MacEachern T, et al.** The use of methylphenidate in patients with incident cancer pain receiving regular opiates: a preliminary report. Pain. 1992;50:75-7.

70. **Forrest WH, Brown BW, Brown CR, et al.** Dextroamphetamine with morphine for the treatment of postoperative pain. N Engl J Med. 1977;296:712-15.

71. **Silverstone T.** The clinical pharmacology of appetite: its relevance to psychiatry. Psychol Med. 1983;13:251-3.

72. **Woods SW, Tesar GE, Murray GB, Cassem EH.** Psychostimulant treatment of depressive disorders secondary to medical illness. J Clin Psychiatry. 1986;47:12-15.

73. **Masand P, Pickett P, Murray GB.** Psychostimulants for secondary depression in medical illness. Psychosomatics. 1991;32:203-8.

74. **Fernandez F, Adams F, Levy JK, et al.** Cognitive impairment due to AIDS-related complex and its response to psychostimulants. Psychosomatics. 1988;29:38-46.

75. **Angrist B, D'Hollosy M, Sanfilipo M, et al.** Central nervous stimulants as symptomatic treatments for AIDS-related neuropsychiatric impairment. J Clin Psychopharmacol. 1992;12:268-72.

76. **Kasper S, Fuger J, Moller H-J.** Comparative efficacy of antidepressants. Drugs. 1992;43(Suppl 2):11-23.

77. **Elliot AJ, Uldall KK, Bergam K, et al.** Randomized, placebo-controlled trial of paroxetine versus imipramine in depressed HIV-positive outpatients. Am J Psychiatry. 1998;153:367-72.

78. **Roose SP, Laghrissi-Thode F, Kennedy JS, et al.** Comparison of paroxetine and nortriptyline in depressed pateints with ischemic heart disease. JAMA. 1998;279:287-91.

79. **Preskorn SH, Burke M.** Somatic therapy for major depressive disorder: selection of an antidepressant. J Clin Psychiatry. 1992;53:(Suppl):5-18.
80. **Mendels J.** Clinical experience with serotonin reuptake inhibiting antidepressants. J Clin Psychiatry. 1987;48:(Suppl):26-30.
81. **Rifkin A, Reardon G, Siris S, et al.** Trimipramine in physical illness with depression. J Clin Psychiatry. 1985;46:4-8.
82. **France RD.** The future for antidepressants: treatment of pain. Psychopathology. 1987;20:99-113.
83. **Preskorn SH, Kerkovich GS.** Central nervous system toxicity of tricyclic antidepressants: phenomenology, course, risk factors, and role of therapeutic drug monitoring. J Clin Psychopharmacol. 1990;10:88-95.
84. **Preskorn SH.** Recent pharmacologic advances in anti-depressant therapy for the elderly. Am J Med. 1993;94:(Suppl):5A.
85. **Lewis Fernandez R, Kleinman A.** Cultural psychiatry: theoretical, clinical and research issues. Psychiatr Clin North Am. 1995;18:433-48.
86. **Farberow M, Ganzler S, Cutter F, Reynolds D.** An eight year survey of hospital suicides. Suicide Life Threat Behav. 1971;1:184-201.
87. **Marzuk PM, Tierney H, Tardiff K, et al.** Increased risk of suicide in persons with AIDS. JAMA. 1988;259:1333-7.
88. **Blazer DG, Bachar JR, Mantor KE.** Suicide in later life: review and commentary. J Am Geriatric Soc. 1986;34:519-25.
89. **Rabins PV.** Prevention of mental disorder in the elderly: current perspectives and future perspectives. J Am Geriatric Soc. 1992;40:727-33.
90. **Ganizini L, Lee MA, Heintz RT, et al.** The effect of depression treatment on elderly patients' preferences for life-sustaining medical therapy. Am J Psychiatry. 1994;151:1631-6.
91. **Block SD, Billings JA.** Patient requests to hasten death: evaluation and management in terminal care. Arch Intern Med. 1994;154:2039-47.
92. **Quill T, Meier D, Block SD, Billings JA.** Physician involvement in hastening death: general principles, data, and disagreement. Ann Intern Med. 1998;128:552-8.
93. **Vachon MLS.** The emotional problems of the patient. In: Doyle D, Hanks GWC, MacDonald N, eds. Oxford Textbook of Palliative Medicine. Oxford: Oxford Medical Publications; 1998.
94. **Endicott J.** Measurement of depression in patients with cancer. Cancer. 1984;53(Suppl):2243-9.
95. **MacKenzie TB, Popkin MK.** Suicide in the medical patient. Intl J Psychiatr Med. 1987;17:3-22.

CHAPTER 7

Diagnosis and Management of Delirium Near the End of Life

DAVID J. CASARETT, MD, MA • SHARON K. INOUYE, MD, MPH

Patients near the end of life may face a variety of symptoms that are distressing and debilitating. Of these, perhaps none is as detrimental to quality of life, and as difficult to diagnose and manage, as delirium. Broadly understood as a disturbance of consciousness, cognition, and perception, with a fluctuating course (1), delirium is a common obstacle to high-quality end-of-life care.

Delirium occurs in 28% to 83% of patients near the end of life, depending on the population studied and the criteria used (2-6). Delirium is a significant problem at the end of life for several reasons. First, delirium may be quite frightening to patients and may cause as much distress as dyspnea, pain, or other symptoms. In addition, families may suffer when the patient, with whom they had hoped to spend meaningful time, is unable to communicate. Finally, the loss of cognitive function robs patients of valuable time and curtails opportunities to make final choices and plans. For all of these reasons, delirium can be a daunting obstacle to good end-of-life care if not addressed appropriately.

The skills required for the diagnosis and management of delirium at the end of life should be a part of every clinician's repertoire. Prompt recognition and appropriate treatment of delirium is a necessary first step to improving patient comfort, optimizing quality of life, and enhancing the leave-taking process for the patient and family. In this paper, we present strategies for the diagnosis and management of delirium near the end of life. We begin by describing a patient who develops mental status changes of uncertain etiology. We give steps for the diagnosis of delirium and evaluation of potential causes and conclude by discussing strategies for prevention and treatment.

Diagnosis of Mental Status Changes

As with all other clinical decisions near the end of life, the patient's and family's goals for care are of central importance. Some patients may wish to preserve their ability to communicate and may be willing to tolerate some degree of discomfort in order to do so. For others, maximizing comfort may be more important. For the former patients diagnostic evaluation and treatment of mental status changes would be appropriate, but for the latter patients any diagnostic or therapeutic interventions should be more circumscribed. Nevertheless, for all patients clinicians should remember that mental status changes are not inevitable. When mental status changes cause distress or when they conflict with the goals of care, they should be treated as aggressively as pain or other symptoms. For all patients, clarifying the goals of care early is necessary in order to provide high-quality care to patients at the end of life.

CASE 7-1. A 42-YEAR-OLD WOMAN WITH OVARIAN CANCER

Mrs. Ghoduay is a 42-year-old woman with ovarian cancer metastatic to peritoneum, liver, and lung. She has become increasingly agitated during the past week, and her husband, daughter, and nurse believe that these changes are caused by pain. However, attempts to increase her opioid dose have resulted in sedation, and she is admitted for evaluation. Her physician, Dr. Marks, finds her to be somnolent and unresponsive to direct questioning. He is unable to assess her pain or other symptoms.

In this case, Dr. Marks should consider the possibility of delirium, which is a syndrome of intermittent alterations in attention, cognition, and perception. Delirium is often obvious, but as many as half of delirium episodes are not noted by clinicians (7,8). Delirium is often missed because it is a clinical diagnosis, which must be made with a careful history, bedside evaluation, and cognitive assessment. In particular, clinicians should note the features of an acute onset, inattention, altered level of consciousness, and cognitive impairment, which are the hallmarks of delirium.

This requires that clinicians have an accurate picture of the patient's baseline cognitive functioning. Therefore Dr. Marks should first inquire about Mrs. Ghoduay's baseline mental status and her mental status at several points in the past. This may require tenacious detective work and questioning of several family members. For instance, Dr. Marks could ask for specific examples of Mrs. Ghoduay's interactions with friends and family a day ago or a week ago. He might also assess her ability to participate in conversations or to recognize family. This line of questioning often proves valuable in defining the time, course, and degree of mental status changes.

> *Further questioning reveals that Mrs. Ghoduay's decline in mental status began approximately 1 week before admission. During the past week, her mental status has fluctuated dramatically, with periods of lucidity punctuated by episodes of somnolence and agitation. During that period, her morphine was increased from 100 mg/24 hr to approximately 400 mg/24 hours, including rescue doses. Her oral intake has been limited. Physical examination reveals no signs that death is imminent. Based on this information, Dr. Marks believes that delirium is a possible cause of her somnolence.*

Evaluating Possible Delirium

To determine whether Mrs. Ghoduay's mental status changes are caused by delirium, Dr. Marks should first search for evidence of cognitive impairment and deficits in attention. Of the tests to assess cognitive function, the Mini Mental Status Examination (MMSE) has the advantage of general availability and familiarity to most clinicians (9).

Therefore, in most settings it should be the test of choice. For assessing attention, the immediate repetition of three objects and the spelling backward (e.g., "d-l-r-o-w") of items can be very useful. Corroboration can be sought in the digit span test, in which inability to repeat at least five numbers forward without errors indicates inattention (10).

These tests support a diagnosis of delirium, but they are not diagnostic. Dr. Marks should also use one of several instruments that have been developed to distinguish delirium from other causes of altered mental status. The most widely used include the Confusion Assessment Method (Table 7-1) (11), the Delirium Rating Scale (12,13), and the Delirium Symptom Interview (14). Each has its own strengths and limitations, and the choice of delirium instruments depends on the goals of use. The Confusion Assessment Method is rapid, easy to use, and validated for identification of delirium by trained clinical and lay interviewers (11) but requires a separate cognitive assessment. On the other hand, the Delirium Rating Scale and the Delirium Symptom Interview are self-contained. The Delirium Rating Scale was designed to be completed after detailed psychiatric assessment and has been validated for use by psychiatrists. The Delirium Symptom Interview has been validated for use by trained clinical and lay interviewers, but its ability to distinguish delirium from dementia has not been adequately tested. Once delirium has been diagnosed, the Delirium Rating Scale or the Memorial Delirium Assessment Scale (15) is valuable for following changes in the severity of delirium symptoms.

Table 7-1. Confusion Assessment Method.

- *Feature 1. Acute Onset and Fluctuating Course*
  Is there evidence of an acute change in mental status from the patient's baseline? Did the (abnormal) behavior fluctuate during the day (e.g., come and go, increase and decrease in severity)?
- *Feature 2. Inattention*
  Did the patient have difficulty focusing attention (e.g., by being easily distracted, or by having difficulty keeping track of what was being said)?
- *Feature 3. Disorganized Thinking*
  Was the patient's thinking disorganized or incoherent (e.g., rambling or irrelevant conversation, unclear or illogical flow of ideas, unpredictable switching from subject to subject)?
- *Feature 4. Altered Level of Consciousness*
  Overall, how would you rate this patient's level of consciousness: alert (normal), vigilant (hyperalert), lethargic (drowsy, easily aroused), stupor (difficult to arouse), or coma (unarousable)?

Mrs. Ghoduay's mental status seemed to improve shortly after admission, and she achieved an MMSE score of 16, but she was unable to perform the serial sevens task or to spell "world" backwards. She was able to repeat only two digits in the digit span test on several occasions. Throughout the interview, Mrs. Ghoduay was easily distracted and often appeared to drift off to sleep. Later the same day, she could be aroused only with difficulty, and attempts to repeat the same tests were unsuccessful.

Characterizing Delirium and Identifying Causes

Based on her clinical course and the results of formal testing, Dr. Marks believes that Mrs. Ghoduay's mental changes are most likely caused by delirium. Delirium may present as one of three major types. The hyperactive or "agitated" delirium, characterized by a hyperaroused state with agitation and hallucinations, is often readily apparent. However, a hypoactive or "quiet" delirium, which is characterized by a decreased level of consciousness with somnolence or stupor, can be mistaken for sedation caused by opioids or obtundation in the last days of life. Finally, a delirium of mixed type, alternating between agitated and quiet forms, may also be difficult to recognize. Of these, Mrs. Ghoduay's presentation is most consistent with a quiet delirium.

Even when delirium is recognized and characterized, an etiology is often elusive because delirium is the product of complex interaction between a vulnerable patient and precipitating factors. Nevertheless, it is important to sift through possible causes to identify those that are easily treatable and that, successfully treated, offer the best chance of improved quality of life (Table 7-2). Once the diagnosis of delirium is made, possible causes can be sought in the medication history, physical examination, and laboratory tests.

Medication History

Data suggest that medication effects are the most common cause of delirium both in the general patient population (7) and in patients near the end of life (4). Several medications commonly used in the palliative care setting deserve emphasis (Table 7-2). Opioids can cause both substantial alterations in mental status (16) and more subtle, temporary changes in cognition and attention (17,18). These changes may become pronounced in the setting of renal failure. There are few data to suggest that one opioid poses a greater risk of delirium than another, but meperidine may have a particularly high risk (19).

A variety of other medications might also be contributors in Mrs. Ghoduay's case (Table 7-2). These include gastrointestinal drugs such as cimetidine, ranitidine, and metoclopramide, as well as many nonsteroidal anti-inflammatory agents and those with prominent anticholinergic effects such as diphenhydramine, hydroxyzine, scopolamine, and amitriptyline (20,21). Corticosteroid psychosis is also a well-described form of delirium related to steroid use.

In evaluating medications, it is also important to consider over-the-counter medications. In addition, the use of complementary medications is quite common, and clinicians may be unaware of their use (22,23). The side effect and interaction profiles of these agents are poorly understood and are difficult to characterize because of variations in formulation and dose. Therefore, questions about comple-

Table 7-2. Contributors to Mental Status Changes Near the End of Life (4,31).

Medical Contributors	Common Medications
Infection	Opioids
Brain metastases	Corticosteroids
Hepatic encephalopathy	Metoclopramide
Renal failure	Benzodiazepines
Hypercalcemia	Hydroxyzine
Hyponatremia	Diphenhydramine
Disseminated intravascular coagulation	NSAIDs
Hypoxemia	H_2 blockers
Volume depletion	Tricyclic antidepressants
Infections (e.g., urinary tract infections, pneumonia)	Scopolamine
Atelectasis with hypoxemia	
Immobilization	

Psychosocial Contributors
Depression
Vision/hearing impairment
Pain
Emotional stress
Unfamiliar environment

mentary and over-the-counter medication use should be part of the medical history.

Identification of a likely medication often suggests a solution. For instance, most medications can be switched to another (e.g., cimetidine and ranitidine) or can be tapered (e.g., corticosteroids). Similarly, in the case of delirium caused by opioids, it is often possible to improve pain relief while improving mental status by rotating to a different opioid at a reduced equianalgesic dose (16,24). This rotation often reduces side effects while maintaining or even improving pain control.

Unfortunately, careful medication review will usually identify several possible contributing drugs. Furthermore, many of the most likely medications may have an important role in pain and symptom management. Because delirium is multifactorial, it is unrealistic to expect that a single medication change will completely resolve the delirium. Instead, clinicians should limit the number of medications whenever possible and substitute agents with more benign side effect profiles.

Physical Examination

Information from a careful history should be supplemented by a physical examination. Some of the most important findings on physical examination are those that indicate a patient is actively dying—hypotension and periods of apnea, for example. The clinician should be alert for signs such as fever, focal neurologic findings, or asterixis. Although the predictive value of these findings in dying patients is not known, their presence can help to guide the diagnostic evaluation. Vision and hearing should be assessed as well because these are important modifiable risk factors for delirium (25).

Clinicians should also be alert to signs of volume depletion, which may be a common cause of delirium near the end of life (4). However, the treatment of volume depletion should not be automatic. Fluid replacement using a nasogastric tube or intravenous catheter may impose additional burdens on the patient and his or her family. Other less invasive interventions such as hypodermoclysis (26) pose fewer burdens. Nevertheless, all of these interventions may prolong the patient's life, which may not be consistent with his or her goals.

Dr. Marks concludes that Mrs. Ghoduay's delirium is caused in part by diphenhydramine that was prescribed for sleep. In addition, he believes that her delirium might be potentiated by high doses of morphine. However, her family is not satisfied with this description. They are concerned about possible metabolic derangements or metastases that might be treatable, and they urge Dr. Marks to pursue a more aggressive evaluation.

Laboratory Evaluation

The decision to search more aggressively for causes of delirium depends on the patient's goals for care, the burdens of an evaluation, and the likelihood that a specific treatable cause will be found. Dr. Marks should also consider the patient's prognosis. Patients who are actively dying frequently experience mental status changes (4,27), and these changes may be resistant to treatment. When death seems to be imminent, it is appropriate to forgo evaluation beyond a history and physical examination and to provide both pharmacologic and non-pharmacologic interventions to ameliorate the symptoms of agitated delirium.

If the clinician and family decide to pursue a diagnostic laboratory or radiologic evaluation, data are not available to dictate a "standard" algorithm. Nevertheless, metabolic causes of delirium are common. In one case series, 18% of terminally ill cancer patients had a metabolic cause of mental status changes (4). Therefore, a targeted laboratory assessment might include complete blood count with differential, electrolytes, blood urea nitrogen, creatinine, calcium, magnesium, phosphorus, glucose, urinalysis, and oxygen saturation. This assessment should be tailored to the individual clinical situation.

The burden of the evaluation, the value of the findings, and the goals of treatment should guide decisions about laboratory or radiologic assessment. The clinical setting must also be considered because treatment of metabolic derangements may be difficult in the home care setting. Therefore, each diagnostic and therapeutic decision requires careful discussion with the patient and his or her family. Evidence of the patient's previous wishes may be particularly helpful in this regard, and it may be helpful to include discussions of treatment options for quiet delirium in early discussions.

Laboratory studies reveal new renal insufficiency but no electrolyte disorder that could explain Mrs. Ghoduay's mental status changes. An oxygen saturation is 93% on 2 L of oxygen by nasal cannula. After a discussion at the bedside, Dr. Marks and Mrs. Ghoduay's family agree to treat her delirium symptomatically.

Dr. Marks recommends a change from morphine to hydromorphone at a reduced equianalgesic dose. On this new regimen, Mrs. Ghoduay's level of consciousness still waxes and wanes and her attention span remains short. She cannot maintain a conversation and drifts off to sleep frequently. Her MMSE scores range from 10 to 15 over 2 days, and her digit span test is between 0 and 2. Her family would like to know if there are other options for symptomatic treatment, even though they realize a cause has not been identified.

Prevention and Treatment

Delirium is often a distressing symptom, like pain, dyspnea, or nausea. Like these symptoms, delirium is treatable. Because patients' time is often limited, clinicians should consider treating delirium before, or in concert with, a diagnostic evaluation. As in pain management, relief of suffering should not be delayed by a search for an etiology of a pain complaint. Instead, the decision to treat the symptoms of pain or delirium should usually be made independently of the results of the etiologic evaluation.

Like pain management, the decision to intervene also depends on the degree to which the symptoms of delirium are distressing. For instance, some patients may experience hallucinations of deceased friends or relatives that appear to be comforting. Families should be reassured that the hallucinations are not a sign of mental illness and do not seem to be distressing to the patient. Nevertheless, the course of delirium is highly variable, and providers should be alert to the development of far more distressing manifestations of delirium.

Prevention and Nonpharmacologic Treatment

All patients near the end of life should be considered at high risk for delirium, and preventive strategies that have been proven effective are indicated for all patients (25). For instance, protocols designed to encourage cognitive activity and to help patients orient to place, time, and environment can be effective. Sleep can be improved by a combination of nonpharmacologic interventions such as relaxation and breathing techniques, quiet music at bedtime, and by reducing environmental light, noise, and other factors that may awaken the patient at night. These strategies offer the significant advantage of minimizing sedative medications, which are a common cause of delirium.

Immobility can be ameliorated in some patients by encouraging out-of-bed time and active range of motion exercises, and by limiting the use of catheters, restraints, or continuous intravenous infusions. All of these factors are potentially modifiable and should be considered not only for prevention but also as potential targets for the nonpharmacologic treatment of delirium. All of these interventions need to be adapted to the individual patient near the end of life and should be consistent with their goals for care.

Pharmacologic Treatment

Several nonpharmacologic interventions are initiated, including careful attention to the lighting in Mrs. Ghoduay's room and orientation cues. In addition, Dr. Marks recommends initiating a trial of haloperidol intravenously, and he explains its efficacy as an antipsychotic. However, Mrs. Ghoduay's family members are reluctant to agree to this plan, arguing that she is not "crazy." The housestaff caring for her also object. They are concerned that haloperidol is not effective treatment for a quiet delirium like Mrs. Ghoduay's and that, if anything, it will only make her more sedated.

In most cases, the goal of pharmacologic treatment of delirium is to bring patients closer to their baseline mental state, not to sedate them or suppress agitation. Therefore, haloperidol should be considered as the first-line therapy for delirium in terminally ill patients (Table 7-3). One randomized controlled trial has shown this agent to be superior to benzodiazepines for both hyperactive and hypoactive delirium (28). Haloperidol has the additional advantages of a fairly wide therapeutic window, availability in both parenteral and oral preparations, and minimal risk of respiratory depression. Although haloperidol is generally safe and effective, it is possible that delirium will initially become worse with treatment. Other important side effects of haloperidol include hypotension and dystonia. Clinicians should be aware of these possibilities and alert family members and other providers to them.

Other agents are available but have fewer data to support their use. Some clinicians have found newer neuroleptics to be effective, including methotrimeprazine, risperidone, clozapine, and olanzapine (see Table 7-3). These agents may offer some advantages over haloperidol, such as diminished extrapyramidal effects (olanzapine, clozapine) and analgesia (methotrimeprazine). However, without data to support their use in the palliative care setting, and without extensive experience in this patient population, these agents should be reserved for use as second-line agents when haloperidol is ineffective.

In some cases, several agents are ineffective, and patients may require sedation. Several authors have suggested that sedation is required in 9% to 26% of patients near the end of life with delirium (27,29). Because sedation may pose its own risks, such as decreased interaction with family or respiratory depression, the decision to use sedation should be weighed carefully against the patient and family's goals for care. For instance, patients with an agitated delirium may experience considerable distress, as may their families. In these cases, therefore, the benefits of sedation may outweigh the risks, given a patient's goals for care (30).

If sedation is warranted, clinicians should choose an agent that is short-acting and easily and rapidly titrated to effect (e.g., lorazepam, midazolam, propofol) (see Table 7-3). Lorazepam is widely used and can be administered by oral, intravenous, and subcutaneous routes; however, it also has the longest duration of action of these drugs.

Table 7-3. Pharmacologic Management of Delirium: Usual Starting Doses of Selected Drugs.

Predominantly Antipsychotic Effects
Haloperidol 0.5-1 mg po q 60 min (0.5-1 mg q 60 min SQ or IV)
Olanzapine 2.5-5 mg po
Risperidone 0.5 mg po bid

Predominantly Sedative Effects
Lorazepam 0.5-1 mg q 4 hr po/IV/SQ
Propofol 10 mg bolus followed by 10 mg/hr IV
Midazolam 1-2 mg/hr IV/SQ

Propofol offers the advantage of rapid titration; however, it is quite expensive and its use is often restricted to the intensive care unit setting or to anesthesiologists. Midazolam may be somewhat more difficult to titrate, but it can be given subcutaneously, although there are limited data to guide dosing by this route. Without convincing data regarding one or the other of these agents, if sedation is necessary, the choice between them should be based on availability and on the requirements of the specific clinical situation.

Summary

Delirium poses a critical challenge to quality of life at the end of life, and adequate identification and management of delirium are essential to good end-of-life care. Nevertheless, this may not be easy. The challenge of providing good treatment for delirium, as with many other symptoms near the end of life, is made more difficult by the paucity of data to guide management decisions. The data that are available come from other patient populations, particularly the elderly (31), and may not be applicable to patients with a variety of diagnoses who are nearing the end of life.

Future research is needed to identify risk factors for delirium that are specific to patients near the end of life. Data are also needed to identify patients for whom laboratory assessment and imaging are likely to be helpful. Finally, data are needed regarding prevention and particularly treatment of delirium in the end-of-life setting. Although this research raises ethical problems related to informed consent, these difficulties are surmountable (32).

Nevertheless, until more data are available, health care providers should be able to identify and effectively manage most cases of delirium using the assessment techniques and interventions outlined here. Establishing goals for care early in the illness course is one of the most important ways to ensure optimal treatment of delirium and other end-of- life symptoms. Although many causes of delirium are easily treated, others require a more intensive evaluation and more aggressive treatment. Preferences regarding goals for treatment, and remaining alert, can be invaluable in guiding these choices.

When delirium occurs, its impact on the patient's quality of life should be assessed. Nonpharmacologic interventions should be used in all cases, with additional pharmacologic therapy if an effect on quality of life is apparent. In all cases, when delirium is distressing to the patient, treatment should be initiated before an evaluation is complete. By safeguarding or restoring cognitive function in these ways, clinicians are laying the foundation for high-quality end-of-life care.

Acknowledgements

Grateful appreciation is offered for the Research Career Development Award in Health Services Research from the Department of Veterans Affairs (DJC) and the Midcareer Award (#K24 AG00949) from the National Institute on Aging and the Donaghue Investigator Award (#DF98-105) from the Patrick and Catherine Weldon Donaghue Medical Research Foundation (SKI).

REFERENCES

1. **American Psychiatric Association.** Diagnostic and Statistical Manual of Mental Disorders (DSM IV), 4th ed. Washington, DC: American Psychiatric Association; 1994.
2. **Massie MJ, Holland J, Glass E.** Delirium in terminally ill cancer patients. Am J Psychiatry. 1983;140:1048-50.
3. **Minagawa H, Uchitomi Y, Yamawaki S, Ishitani K.** Psychiatric morbidity in terminally ill cancer patients. Cancer. 1996;78:1131-7.
4. **Bruera E, Miller L, McCallion J, et al.** Cognitive failure in patients with terminal cancer: a prospective study. J Pain Symptom Manage. 1992;7:192-5.
5. **Leipzig RM, Goodman H, Gray G, et al.** Reversible, narcotic-associated mental status impairment in patients with metastatic cancer. Pharmacology. 1987;35:47-54.
6. **Pereira J, Hanson J, Bruera E.** The frequency and clinical course of cognitive impairment in patients with terminal cancer. Cancer. 1997;79:835-42.
7. **Francis J, Strong S, Martin D, Kapoor W.** Delirium in elderly general medical patients: common but often unrecognized. Clin Res. 1988;36:711A.
8. **Gustafson Y, Brannstrom B, Norberg A, et al.** Underdiagnosis and poor documentation of acute confusional states in elderly hip fracture patients. J Am Geriatr Soc. 1991;39:760-5.
9. **Folstein MF, Folstein F, McHugh PR.** "Mini-mental state": a practical method for grading the cognitive state of patients for the clinician. J Psych Res. 1975;12:189-98.
10. **Pompei P, Foreman M, Cassel CK, et al.** Detecting delirium among hospitalized older patients. Arch Intern Med. 1995;155:301-7.
11. **Inouye SK, van Dyck CH, Alessi CA.** Clarifying confusion: the Confusion Assessment Method, a new method for detection of delirium. Ann Intern Med. 1990;113:941-8.

12. **Trzepacz PT, Baker RW, Greenhouse J.** A symptom rating scale for delirium. Psych Res. 1988;23:89-97.

13. **Trzepacz PT, Dew MA.** Further analyses of the Delirium Rating Scale. Gen Hosp Psych. 1995;17:75-9.

14. **Albert MS, Levkoff SE, Reilly C, et al.** The Delirium Symptom Interview: an interview for the detection of delirium symptoms in hospitalized patients. J Geriatr Psychiatry Neurol. 1992;5:14-21.

15. **Breitbart W, Rosenfeld B, Roth A, et al.** The Memorial Delirium Assessment Scale. J Pain Symptom Manage. 1997;13:128-37.

16. **de Stoutz ND, Bruera E, Suarez-Almazor M.** Opioid rotation for toxicity reduction in terminal cancer patients. J Pain Symptom Manage. 1995;10:378-84.

17. **Bruera E, MacMillan K, Kuchn N, et al.** The cognitive effects of the administration of narcotics. Pain. 1989;39:13-16.

18. **Wood M, Ashby M, Somogyi A, Fleming B.** Neuropsychological and pharmacokinetic assessment of hospice inpatients receiving morphine. J Pain Symptom Manage. 1998;16:112-20.

19. **Marcantonio ER, Juarez G, Goldman L, et al.** The relationship of postoperative delirium with psychoactive medications. JAMA. 1994;272:1518-22.

20. **Gustafson Y, Berggen D, Brannstrom B, et al.** Acute confusional states in elderly patients treated for femoral fracture. J Am Geriatr Soc. 1988;36:525-30.

21. **Schor JD, Levkoff SE, Lipsitz L, et al.** Risk factors for delirium in hospitalized elderly. JAMA. 1992;267:827-31.

22. **Paramore LC.** Use of alternative therapies: estimates from the 1994 Robert Wood Johnson Foundation National Access to Care Survey. J Pain Symptom Manage. 1997;13:83-9.

23. **Burstein HJ, Gelber S, Weeks JC.** Use of alternative medicine by women with early-stage breast cancer. N Engl J Med. 1999;340:1733-9.

24. **Bruera E, Franco JJ, Maltoni M, et al.** Changing pattern of agitated impaired mental status in patients with advanced cancer: association with cognitive monitoring, hydration, and opioid rotation. J Pain Symptom Manage. 1995;10:287-91.

25. **Inouye S, Bogardus ST, Charpentier PA, et al.** A multicomponent intervention to prevent delirium in hospitalized older patients. N Engl J Med. 1999;340:669-76.

26. **Steiner N, Bruera E.** Methods of hydration in palliative care patients. J Pall Care. 1998;14:6-13.

27. **Fainsinger R, MacEachern T, Hanson J, et al.** Symptom control during the last week of life in a palliative care unit. J Pall Care. 1991;7:5-11.

28. **Breitbart W, Marotta R, Platt MM, et al.** A double-blind trial of haloperidol, chlorpromazine, and lorazepam in the treatment of delirium in hospitalized AIDS patients. Am J Psych. 1996;153:231-7.

29. **Ventafridda V, Ripamonti C, DeConno F, et al.** Symptom prevalence and control during cancer patients' last days of life. J Pall Care. 1990;6:7-11.

30. **Quill TE, Byock IR.** Responding to intractable suffering: the role of terminal sedation and voluntary refusal of food and fluids. Ann Intern Med. 2000;132:408-14.
31. **Inouye SK, Charpentier PA.** Precipitating factors for delirium in hospitalized elderly persons: predictive model and interrelationship with baseline vulnerability. JAMA. 1996;275:852-7.
32. **Casarett D, Karlawish J.** Are special ethical guidelines needed for palliative care research? J Pain Symptom Manage. 2000;20:130-9.

CHAPTER 8

Dying Patients in the Intensive Care Unit: Forgoing Treatment and Maintaining Care

KATHY FABER-LANGENDOEN, MD • PAUL N. LANKEN, MD

U p to 60% of deaths in the United States occur in acute care hospitals (1); of these deaths, 75% to 80% occur after decisions to forgo treatment (2,3). Among all Medicare enrollees, 31% are admitted to an intensive care unit (ICU) within 6 months of death (4). Explicit decisions to forgo treatment are commonplace, but despite improvements brought about by public education, prominent court cases, and palliative care curricula, the care of patients dying in ICUs continues to raise clinical and ethical difficulties. In a survey of nurses and physicians, 55% believed that patients are sometimes overburdened by the treatments given them (5). More than half believed that mechanical ventilators, cardiopulmonary resuscitation, and dialysis were often used inappropriately. The SUPPORT study included number of days spent in the ICU as one indicator of poor outcome, indicating at least ambivalence about the place of the ICU in the care of the dying (6).

Certainly the ICU poses challenges to the care of the dying. Recognizing that treatment is not working or is not meeting the patient's objectives involves dramatic shifts in an ICU oriented towards the rescue of patients from life-threatening conditions. Decisions in the ICU may be more complex than in other units in the hospital. Patients are often unable to participate in decisions because of sedation or the severity of illness. Consultants may give conflicting information and potentially slow decision-making as each is consulted. And, if a decision to limit treatment is made, clinicians are faced with multiple drugs, technologies, and assessments, any or all of which could be discontinued, without a clear sense of how to proceed. Will stopping a ventilator make an agitated patient more or less comfortable? Is it better to stop something that quickly leads to death (e.g., vasopressors), or ought one choose something with more delayed effects (e.g., dialysis)? Is continued cardiac monitoring distracting, or does it provide useful information? Finally, the ICU's environment, with constant lighting, steady foot traffic, and competition for space between machines and people, is not conducive to caring for dying patients and their families.

On the other hand, ICUs present certain advantages in providing humane care of the dying. Highly trained ICU nurses who spend extended hours with a given patient and family facilitate an understanding of family dynamics and concerns. ICUs provide medical and nursing resources unavailable in other settings that can be used to care for seriously ill patients, including some of those who are dying. The seriousness of the patient's illness often brings together family members who can help articulate patient values and wishes and provide evidence of the patient's community. Furthermore, ICUs affiliated with academic centers provide venues for professional education and clinical research that could elucidate clinical issues in the care of the dying.

This paper aims to help clinicians navigate the care of ICU patients for whom a decision has been made to limit life-sustaining treatment. The case presented (based on an actual case, with personal and identifying information altered to protect privacy) shows some of the difficulties clinicians face, including the relevance of prognostic models, decision-making in the context of cultural and religious differences, and the clinical management of the process of forgoing specific interventions. It challenges the misconception that such decisions are decisions to withdraw care (7) and encourages physicians to approach the care of these patients with the same attention to detail, critical thinking, and compassion that accompanies the care of ICU patients expected to survive.

CASE 8-1. A 79-YEAR-OLD MALE ADMITTED WITH ACUTE ABDOMINAL PAIN

Mr. McGee is a 79-year-old retired minister who is admitted with acute abdominal pain. He had been in good health except for complete heart block requiring pacemaker placement 3 years ago. He lived at home and cared for his wife, who was severely disabled from rheumatoid arthritis. The day after admission, he developed a perforated bowel and was taken for surgical repair. His postoperative course in the ICU was complicated by acute respiratory distress syndrome that required mechanical ventilation and by candidal peritonitis and acute renal failure that necessitated dialysis. His condition deteriorated during the 3 weeks after surgery. He was no longer able to engage in conversations or follow commands, although he seemed intermittently aware of his family's presence.

Mr. McGee's family was told by the ICU attending physician that his chances for recovering his prehospital level of function were nil and that, even with all available measures, his chance of surviving this hospitalization was less than 10%. Furthermore, they were told that the best that could be hoped was eventual discharge to a nursing home, where he would almost certainly need long-term ventilator support and dialysis. Although the patient had no written advance directive, Mrs. McGee and their son were certain that Mr. McGee would not want to continue this kind of life, given his belief in an afterlife and statements he had made during the last year that he was "ready to be with the Lord."

Use and Limits of Prognostication

Substantial advances have been made in providing objective, statistically based predictions of hospital mortality for ICU patients. Several regression models have been developed to predict hospital mortality of ICU patients and are useful tools in determining outcomes of large groups of patients (8-10). To what extent can these predictions reduce prognostic uncertainty and inform end-of-life care for individual patients like Mr. McGee? To assess this, consider the questions discussed in the following sections.

Will the Patient Live or Die?

When families ask if their loved one will survive, they would like a "yes" or "no" answer rather than a probability of survival. Only rarely can the ICU physician honestly respond in such a manner. Prognostic models cannot answer "yes" or "no" even for the patient in the highest decile of predicted mortality. Even disease-specific and context-specific models that identify subsets with 100% mortality (e.g., bone marrow transplant patients on ventilators with specific complications of a specified duration) cannot statistically exclude a small chance of survival (11). Thus, the best information that can be truthfully offered is a probability of survival with and without various treatments.

Available prognostic models have other limitations. First, the accuracy of a model's predicted risk of death depends on whether the patient's medical condition reasonably falls within the range of illness severity upon which the model was based. In addition, most ICU prognostic models are derived from prognostic factors present upon ICU admission and do not provide updated mortality estimates while the patient remains in the ICU. Most models also ignore elements reflecting the process of care and the patient's response to that care. Finally, some patients follow inherently unpredictable courses. For example, in one study, the probability of patients with severe congestive heart failure surviving two more months was 62% one day before they died (although most of these patients were hospitalized outside of the ICU) (12).

How Long Will the Patient Survive If He or She Leaves the Hospital Alive?

Conventional ICU prognostic models do not use survival-after-discharge data from the ICU as an outcome. The prognostic model developed specifically for use in SUPPORT provided 2-month and 6-month estimates of survival to patients, families, and ICU physicians, but this information appeared to have minimal impact on the care of those with serious illness (6).

If the Patient Survives, What Will His or Her Quality of Life Be?

No standard ICU prognostic model incorporates quality of life as an outcome, and few data are available to answer this.

Given these limitations, would sophisticated ICU prognostic models have helped decision-making for Mr. McGee? Most clinicians incorporate some form of probabilistic reasoning in discussing prognosis and its inherent uncertainty with patients and families. Having objective estimates of survival may be useful to complement this process. However, current ICU prognostic models should not be relied upon as the sole basis for individual end-of-life decisions. Their availability may help "plant the seed" in the minds of some families that their loved one may actually die in the ICU. From this simple beginning may grow the mutual trust and a more collaborative approach to care in the ICU.

The Process of Decision-Making

Making medical decisions at the end of life is not unique to the ICU setting and has been extensively discussed in several excellent reviews and statements of professional organizations (13,14,17). ICUs, with critically ill patients, stressed families, and multiple consultants, pose particular challenges to decision-making. The tendency of consultants to focus on a single area of expertise may become an obstacle to keeping in view the patient's overall well-being. Multiple consultants provide a barrage of information to families and patients, some of which may conflict with information from other sources. Frequent changes of ICU attendings further threatens strategic planning of patient care. In such an arena, it is essential that a single physician be identified who is responsible for overseeing the patient's care, coordinating and sifting through consultants' recommendations, and ensuring that the patient's well-being and wishes remain the central concerns. If the physician assuming this role will be rotating off service and cannot continue overseeing the patient's care, he or she should directly tell the patient/family who will assume this role and discuss the strategy of care with the new physician. Multiple handoffs such as this within a week create problems that are almost impossible to overcome.

Patients with Decision-Making Capacity

The ethical basis of forgoing life-sustaining treatment resides in the patient's legal and ethical right to determine what should happen to one's own body. An adult patient with the capacity to make the decision at hand must be informed of the options and their possible outcomes. Patients with decisional capacity who decide to forgo life-sustaining treatment should have these decisions honored by their physicians and other clinicians. As a rule, a patient's considered decision should override contrary opinions of a spouse, parents, children, or physicians, no matter how well intentioned and rational the latter may be.

Patients Without Decision-Making Capacity

Upon admission Mr. McGee was competent, and conversations about his wishes should complications arise may have proved useful to his family and physicians later. However, as was the case with Mr. McGee, 60% to 70% of patients are unable to speak for themselves when they are seriously ill and decisions to limit treatment are considered (3,15). Advance directives were devised to enable patients to specify in advance the treatment limits they desire. The absence of a formal advance directive in this case is typical, as generally (with rare exceptions [16]) only 10% to 20% of patients complete advance directives. A growing body of evidence suggests that patients with advance directives may not receive substantially different care from those without such directives. As such, advance directives have been of relatively limited assistance (17).

In the ICU, many family members may gather around the patient. In the absence of a proxy decision-maker previously designated in an advance directive, identifying a single surrogate decision-maker (or, if decisions are made by consensus within the family, a single spokesperson) is helpful. The surrogate should be an adult who knows the patient well and is willing to take on the responsibility to join with the ICU team in shared decision-making on the patient's behalf. The basis for decision-making, in order of preference, is 1) the patient's previously stated preferences regarding end-of-life treatment, 2) inferences based on the patient's values or goals, and 3) weighing the benefits and burdens of treatment in determining what is in the patient's best interests.

In the absence of a proxy or surrogate chosen by the patient, some states or institutional policies designate proxies using a hierarchy similar to that used in determining inheritance of property in the absence of a will or granting permission for an autopsy. At times, the legally mandated and the ethically appropriate person are not the same (e.g., an adult daughter may be a more ethically appropriate surrogate than an estranged wife; a homosexual partner may be a better choice than a parent). For this reason we recommend that all patients, both as part of routine health care and on admission to ICUs, be strongly urged to advise caregivers as to how to make decisions, including designating a health care proxy for medical decisions. Some states do not have legal provisions for health care proxy designation; given the various ways in which states address decision-making for patients without decisional capacity, care should be taken that the process of decision-making does not conflict with laws of the applicable jurisdiction.

ICU clinicians should guide the proxy or surrogate through the decision-making process, keeping in mind their emotional state in response to critical illness. Information should be given using simple terms, avoiding jargon, with ample time for questions and discussion, recognizing the possible need for repeated conversations to help the family absorb the information. In many cases, it is helpful to hold care conferences in which ICU clinicians, the primary care physician, and other consultants meet with the patient (if able), patient's family, close friends, religious advisor, and/or proxy or surrogate (if not one of above). For patients expected to remain in the ICU more than 2 days, these meetings should be held within 48 hours of admission to the ICU. Goals of ICU care should be identified and regularly reassessed. Conferences should be repeated at regular intervals to reassess goals of care in view of the patient's changing medical prognosis. Questions of whether it is still appropriate to continue aggressive, rescue-type ICU interventions need to be addressed in an empathetic and open discussion. Even if the prognosis is as bad and as certain as medical science can "prove" (11,18), many families need time to cope with the rapidity of their loved one's deterioration and the prospect of the patient's death. Dealing with families' sense of loss and emotional issues emphasizes the need for a multi-disciplinary approach to case conferences. Spiritual and religious concerns are often of great significance to patients and families when confronted by serious illness. Nurses and physicians uncomfortable in addressing these issues must, at minimum, inquire as to their importance to the patient and family and find the necessary resources to address these issues. Chaplains and spiritual leaders can often help ensure that spiritual needs are met while patients are in the ICU.

Cultural Variations in Deciding to Forgo Treatment

Physicians should be aware of cultural differences in approaching decisions at the end of life. Recent studies suggest that, in the United States, members from cultures other than the dominant European-American culture may be less willing to discuss resuscitation status (19), less likely to forgo life-sustaining treatment (19-21), and more reluctant to complete advance directives (22,23). The reasons for these differences are only partially understood but may include different cultural and religious values (e.g., rejection of the concept of seeing the patient as the ultimate decision-maker) and distrust of the American health care system or physicians (24). Cultural and religious sensitivity and a willingness to listen to different perspectives are essential attributes of ICU staff. Developing and utilizing the cultural diversity among staff reflecting the patient population may increase an ICU's ability to understand these differences and to provide better care for patients and their families.

A "Do Not Resuscitate" order was written. Taking Mr. McGee home to die was not an option, given his wife's disabilities. The family decided to stop the patient's dialysis. The ICU attending suggested that, in addition, the ventilator be discontinued, and the family agreed the following day.

Before discontinuation of ventilator support, vasopressors, laboratory blood draws, and all medications except morphine and midazolam were discontinued. Enteral feedings were also discontinued by the resident but restarted an hour later at the attending's request.

The Process of Forgoing Life-Sustaining Treatment

The care of Mr. McGee confronted his physicians and family with many decisions. What was the best place to care for him? Which interventions should be continued and which stopped? Ought "artificial nutrition" be dealt with differently than other medical interventions? Decisions to forgo life-sustaining treatment may occur as a single, complete reassessment and change in direction, or may evolve over time, with a gradual stripping away of treatments. In either case, decisions to forgo treatment in the ICU are inherently complex, with multiple medications, interventions, and diagnostic tests usually in use (25).

The frequency and nature of withdrawing treatment in ICUs has undergone substantial evolution in the past 20 years. Withdrawing ventilators was uncommon in 1983, when the first recommendations for discontinuing ventilator support were published (26). During the next 15 years, the rates of decisions not to resuscitate and of withdrawing dialysis, ventilators, and other interventions have increased (27,28). A prospective study recorded treatment limitations among all patients admitted to 136 ICUs. Among 5910 patients dying in these ICUs, 74% had some form of treatment withheld or withdrawn before death. However, interinstitutional variation was large, with individual units reporting anywhere from 21% to 96% of deaths being preceded by limitations of treatment, and some institutions reporting no instances of life support being withdrawn. This remarkable variation among ICUs was largely unexplained, except that patients in New York and Missouri, where laws stipulate "clear and convincing" evidence of patient wishes, were less likely to have treatment withdrawn (2). The extent of this variation raises serious questions as to what extent these practice differences represent variations in physician or institutional values that ignore or override patient wishes.

Withdrawing Multiple Interventions

Mr. McGee's case is typical in that, at the time the decision to forgo treatment was made, multiple interventions (ventilator, dialysis, cardiac monitoring, pacemaker, laboratory analyses, enteral feedings, vasopressors) were in use. In a study of the process of treatment withdrawal in four U.S. hospitals, an average of 3.8 treatments were forgone for each dying patient (25). Of note in Mr. McGee's case, not all life-sustaining treatments were stopped simultaneously, enteral feedings were restarted at the attending physician's request (suggesting ambivalence about stopping artificial feedings that did not extend to stopping the ventilator), and no apparent consideration was given to stopping the pacemaker until he died.

When multiple interventions are in use, a somewhat predictable order of forgoing treatment often ensues, with dialysis, further diag-

nostic workups, and vasopressors being forgone early; intravenous fluids, transfusions, monitoring, laboratory tests, and antibiotics being forgone later; and artificial feedings (enteral and parenteral feedings) and
ventilators being withdrawn last (25). The reasons for this "stepwise
retreat" are complex and may include the relative burdens of the specific interventions, symbolic import of some of the interventions (e.g.,
artificial feeding) to family or clinicians, and immediacy of the effects
of withdrawing a specific intervention. In addition, physicians may be
less likely to withdraw treatments begun to treat iatrogenic problems
or longstanding interventions and more willing to withdraw therapies
related to their own subspecialty (29,30).

In addition to physician biases, patients' surrogates or proxies may
hesitate to stop a mechanical ventilator and let their loved one die as
a result of that decision. They may find it easier to endorse not starting new interventions or withholding antibiotics, blood products, or
vasopressors, where the link between forgoing the intervention and the
patient's death is not so uncomfortably obvious. However, family decision-making about treatment withdrawal remains largely unstudied.

In considering the array of interventions that might be withheld or
withdrawn, we recommend that the focus be on clearly articulating the
goals of care. Even in the setting of treatment withdrawal, goals vary
considerably. Occasionally, the goal may be to remove a particular
treatment perceived to be burdensome (e.g., a ventilator that impairs
communication and separates patient from family). Short-term survival
goals until important loved ones gather may argue for continued ventilator support. Maintaining the ability to communicate means that
vasopressors to maintain blood pressure might be indicated, whereas
if comfort is the primary goal, vasopressors are not beneficial.

Sometimes a specific treatment is not itself burdensome, but the
array of ICU care maintains a life that, in its dependency and suffering,
is so. In such cases, the goals of care may suggest a process in which
interventions are withdrawn in such a way that dying is not prolonged.
A stepwise retreat extending over a few days and slow terminal weans
needlessly prolong the dying process. Although precipitous decisions
do not serve the family's needs well, prolonging dying by slowly titrating away interventions prolongs patient and family suffering and
spends health care dollars with no benefit. We recommend that the
specific goals of continued care for the patient be clearly specified and
agreed upon, after which clinicians assess each intervention, diagnos-

tic test, and medication in light of whether each contributes to achieving the desired goal(s). Interventions that do not contribute to the patient's goals, regardless of whether they are burdensome in their own right, should be discontinued as extraneous to the patient's care. Throughout this process, explicit attention should be paid to measures that will ease the patient's dying and provide comfort, as well as facilitating the completion of important life tasks (e.g., reconciliation with estranged family) as much as is possible in these critically ill patients. Experts in palliative care are often helpful in optimizing such care.

Forgoing Specific Interventions

Enteral and Parenteral Feedings

The clinical and ethical issues surrounding decisions to discontinue artificial nutrition are not unique to the ICU and have been discussed extensively elsewhere (31-34). In Mr. McGee's case, restarting enteral feedings did not contribute to his overall comfort or prolong his life in the setting of ventilator withdrawal. Enteral feedings should not have been restarted unless the family wanted them continued. Some families may find symbolic benefits from continued feeding irrespective of nutritional benefits (35). Although attempts at oral feeding were not possible in Mr. McGee's case given his ventilator dependence, patients able to swallow without risk of aspirating ought to be offered fluids and food as part of comfort care.

Dialysis

Dialysis for critically ill patients is associated with a high mortality, particularly among patients with other serious comorbidities (36). As was the case with Mr. McGee, decisions to discontinue dialysis in the ICU are frequently made in the context of forgoing other life-sustaining treatment.

Unlike withdrawal of a ventilator, stopping dialysis is unlikely to cause death immediately. In a small case series of patients who discontinued chronic hemodialysis, median survival was 9.6 days, with a range of 2 to 34 days (37). When dialysis is initiated for acute renal failure, stopping dialysis may be accompanied by recovery of adequate renal function, and patients and families ought to be prepared for this possibility. Symptoms accompanying the cessation of dialysis may include dyspnea, pruritis, pain, and mental status changes. Dyspnea from volume overload can be minimized by restricting fluids, administering opiates, and, rarely, the use of ultrafiltration. Pruritis may be minimized by application of emollients and use of oral antihistamines. Nausea from uremia may be palliated with phenothiazines or butyrophenones, which are somewhat sedating and may have beneficial effects in treating coexistent mental confusion (38).

Mr. McGee had been receiving infusions of morphine at 8 mg/hr and midazolam at 4 mg/hr for the past 2 weeks in the ICU. Just before ventilator withdrawal, extra boluses of 4 mg of morphine and 2 mg of midazolam were given. The ventilator rate was turned down from 20 to 10, FiO$_2$ decreased to room air, and tidal volume decreased to 600. Mr. McGee's respiratory rate increased to 26; although there were no outward signs of discomfort, the resident increased the ventilator rate to 20 and the tidal volume to 750.

Mechanical Ventilation

Although the ultimate outcome of ventilator withdrawal is virtually always the same (i.e., the patient's death), methods of withdrawing the ventilators vary greatly among physicians and specialists (39).

Some ICU practitioners advocate "terminal weaning," in which the assistance in breathing and the supplemental oxygen provided by the ventilator is gradually reduced. The endotracheal tube (or its equivalent) is left in place during this process. Its proponents believe this approach provides time for the family and ICU staff to adjust to the imminence of the patient's death and "emotional distance" between writing the order to withdraw and the effects of that order (40). Other advocates believe this method allows optimal control of the process and best ensures patient comfort (39,41). However, terminal weaning may misleadingly seem to imply the possibility of successful weaning and it unnecessarily prolongs dying process (42,43).

Other ICU clinicians utilize extubation and removal from mechanical ventilation as their standard of care. Extubation directly and most quickly removes what may be perceived as burdensome treatment.

This approach demands that the staff anticipate and form a strategy for dealing with dyspnea that is likely to accompany cessation of ventilatory support. Extubation has the advantage of allowing death to come quickly. Extubation may cause family distress if the patient's respiratory secretions are voluminous or if the patient develops agonal breathing misinterpreted as reflecting discomfort rather than the dying process, although family perceptions of ventilator withdrawal remain unstudied.

Still another group of ICU specialists promote removing the patient from the ventilator while leaving the airway in place. This allows the staff to keep the airway suctioned but precludes any possibility of verbal communication and may be perceived as "unnatural" or disfiguring by families.

Which technique is better is a question that calls for critical examination of practices currently driven by tradition and emotion. In Mr. McGee's case, a single decrease in ventilatory support was made with only slight increases in opioids and benzodiazepines. As he became tachypneic, even without evidence of discomfort, the ventilator support was increased again. The family had expected the ventilator to be withdrawn so Mr. McGee could die; meanwhile, the resident expected that a single decrease in support was all that would be necessary and had no plans past the initial decrease. Regardless of the method used, it is incumbent upon the ICU physician in charge to formulate a plan and time course for the process of withdrawal, not merely to make a single decrease in ventilator settings expecting that death will rapidly ensue. If physicians choose the more medicalized process of terminal weaning, they must frequently assess the patient's response, respond with appropriate palliative measures, and have a time course in mind for weaning. Prolonged weans lasting more than a few hours have no justification and only prolong dying. Families should be prepared for the possibility that up to 10% of patients may survive more than a few hours after ventilator withdrawal, despite the previous expectation that they will die (44).

The occurrence of dyspnea should be anticipated with ventilator withdrawal by any method. Opiates for dyspnea and discomfort, as well as benzodiazepines for anxiety or agitation, should be immediately available. These drugs may be given to treat documented symptoms or prevent anticipated symptoms from occurring, because the clinician's primary duty in this setting is to ensure patient comfort. The paramount intent of medication in this setting is to alleviate and prevent the distress that often accompanies ventilator withdrawal, not to hasten the patient's death. Intravenous infusions provide the most rapid response, but if intravenous access is not available, subcutaneously administered opiate infusions are also effective. The amount necessary to relieve symptoms varies tremendously among patients depending on previous drug exposure, metabolism, and level of awareness; typical doses of morphine range from 10 to 30 mg/hr, although occasional opioid-tolerant patients have received doses an order of magnitude higher. Physicians and nurses ought to document that medications are being given and increased to relieve symptoms and ensure comfort. The focus of care should be on relieving the patient's discomfort, regardless of the amount of medication needed to accomplish this.

Paralysis caused by neuromuscular blocking agents precludes the assessment of patient discomfort and makes it impossible for patients to communicate with loved ones. For these reasons, neuromuscular blocking agents should be avoided when withdrawing ventilators. They ought never be given to merely make the patient "appear" comfortable. Paralytics already in use should be stopped before ventilator withdrawal and given time to clear or, if possible, pharmacologically reversed (39,45). In the unusual case where effects of these agents persist beyond several hours, physicians should discuss with families the appropriateness of proceeding with ventilator withdrawal, given that such patients remain at risk for unrecognized pain and discomfort (46).

Pacemakers and Implantable Defibrillators

Although Mr. McGee had a pacemaker in place, no apparent consideration was given to deactivating the pacemaker when the decision was made to forgo life-sustaining treatment. Although temporary pacemakers are more likely to elicit such considerations, a permanent pacemaker often goes unnoticed during the process of treatment withdrawal. Pacemakers, once implanted, rarely cause the patient discomfort. However, if a patient wishes to refuse all life-sustaining treatment, even treatments which are not directly burdensome, there is no principled reason not to honor the patient's refusal of further pacemaker treatment, as long as standards for valid decision-making are met (47,48). Similarly, just as patients have the right to refuse attempts at cardiopulmonary resuscitation, they also may decline continued defibrillation as administered by an implantable defibrillator. The outcome of deactivating pacemakers cannot be easily predicted because of difficulty in predicting what intrinsic rhythm may be recovered after the pacemaker is deactivated.

Locations for the Care of Patients Forgoing Life-Sustaining Treatment

The best location for ICU patients who are dying should be explicitly assessed. Transfer to a general ward or a dedicated palliative care or hospice unit may provide excellent care to the patient and family, although transfer may disrupt relationships established between ICU clinicians and patients or families. Some institutions have palliative care units for patients being withdrawn from life-sustaining treatment, allowing a level of expertise unattainable in less specialized settings (41). Remaining in the ICU allows continuity of nursing care, but may do so at prohibitive cost. If dying patients remain in the ICU because of the level of care required, the critical care staff need specific training to become adept in shifting from "rescue medicine" to palliative care techniques. Acquiring these skills requires substantial institutional commitment to necessary training. The optimum location for the care of dying patients who have been in the ICU will vary among institutions, depending on the expertise and organization of patient care. Efforts to maintain continuity with key health care professionals (at minimum, the primary attending and, if possible, the primary nurse) should be made.

When the ICU continues to be the best available place for the dying patient, careful attention should be paid to the ICU environment (49). People often prefer to die at home (50). Although this is impossible for most ICU patients, what aspects of "home" can be simulated in the ICU in order to best care for dying patients and their families?

First, "home" represents privacy for the patient and his or her loved ones during their final days together. ICUs should provide private rooms for dying patients. Activities outside of the patient's room can be readily separated from those inside by utilizing closed doors and curtains to promote privacy. Second, "home" allows family and friends ready access into the dying patient's world. Allowing equivalent access in ICUs requires suspending restrictive visiting policies. Comfortable chairs, recliners, and roll-away cots should be provided to support the family's desire to be with the patient. Third, "home" provides access to the patient's own possessions and amenities, such as favorite music, religious icons, furniture, clothes, pets, food, and drink. No ICU environment can duplicate the patient's world in toto, but transportable elements desired by the patient can be brought to the ICU by family and friends to promote patient comfort. Finally, dying at home often incorporates the assistance of friends and family as personal caregivers. When appropriate to the patient's situation, allowing family and friends to help with patient care provides meaningful and important roles for loved ones.

> *A half hour into the terminal weaning, the family discussed among themselves what would happen to the pacer when Mr. McGee died, and how they would know he was dead with the pacer still firing. After two hours, the son asked "How low does the blood pressure have to go for it to be over?" and after another hour and a half, said "Enough is enough; it's time to stop." The resident was contacted and decreased the ventilator rate to 15 and discontinued the PEEP.*
>
> *Two hours later, Mr. McGee's oxygen saturation and blood pressure fell precipitously. His blood pressure became unobtainable, though the monitor continued to show a paced rhythm at 80. The cardiology fellow was called; arriving 15 minutes later, he disabled the pacemaker. The monitor showed ventricular fibrillation, and Mr. McGee was declared dead.*

During the course of Mr. McGee's ventilator withdrawal, the family was left alone with the nurse to wait for death, with no one else available to provide emotional or spiritual support. An overwhelming sense of personal loss and associated emotional and spiritual suffering are often at the core of a dying person's and family's experience (51). Although ICU nurses and physicians usually are not experts in bereavement, religion and spirituality, or pastoral care, these aspects of caring must not be ignored. The willingness to listen and acknowledge another person's fears, emotions, or spiritual pain is of value. In feeling heard, a suffering person's sense of isolation is diminished. Patients in the ICU should be proactively evaluated for an interest and desire to receive counseling and pastoral care. Chaplains, social workers, counselors, and others skilled in supporting people through personal loss and emotional distress are invaluable resources to the ICU team. Spiritual care may include religious rituals meaningful to the patient and family.

Mr. McGee's family relied on cardiac monitoring and vital signs to gauge the trajectory of his dying, although such monitoring is relatively useless in assessing comfort or accurately predicting time course. When Mr. McGee died, his death was apparently not even accepted by the medical team until the pacemaker was deactivated, providing a technological "last rites" of sorts. At several points during the process of withdrawal, the resident was left alone to deal with technological issues without a clear plan in how to proceed. When Mr. McGee became tachypneic after the initial ventilator decrease, the resident increased the ventilator support back towards the original settings. The resident had no plan as to how to further decrease ventilator support, despite the family's and staff's decision to withdraw. And, rather than turning off the monitor during the process of withdrawal or immediately after the patient had died, the resident mistakenly acted as though Mr. McGee were still alive until the pacemaker was deactivated. All of these actions speak tellingly of the need for expert guidance from experienced clinicians, with the same attention to clinical detail and treatment planning that accompanies the treatment of critical illnesses. One cannot presume that physicians instinctively know how to go about withdrawing treatment, much less that they will instinctively know how to palliate patient symptoms or address emotional or spiritual issues.

Summary

The care of patients dying in the ICU often requires a dramatic shift from the "rescue" mode to approaches that recognize the inevitability of the patient's death and focus on patient and family comfort. Such a shift requires reaching consensus with the patient or family about the goals of ICU care and having a well-developed plan and the clinical skills and knowledge to meet the physical, emotional, and spiritual needs of dying patients and their families. Such skills must not be assumed but can be learned through formal education programs and by positive role-modeling. Further research into decision-making, family and patient values at the end of life, and clinical outcomes beyond survival, including comfort and quality of dying, will help equip ICU clinicians to better meet these challenges.

REFERENCES

1. **Field MJ, Cassel C, eds.** Approaching Death: Improving Care at the End of Life.Washington, DC: National Academy Press; 1997:33-49.
2. **Prendergast TJ, Claessens MT, Luce JM.** A national survey of end-of-life care for critically ill patients. Am J Resp Crit Care Med. 1998;158:1163-7.
3. **Faber-Langendoen K.** A multi-institutional study of care given to patients dying in hospitals: ethical and practice implications. Arch Intern Med. 1996; 156:2130-6.
4. **Wennberg JE, Cooper MM, eds.** The Dartmouth Atlas of Health Care in the United States. Chicago: American Hospital Publishing; 1998:106.
5. **Solomon MZ, O'Donnell L, Jennings B, et al.** Decisions near the end of life: professional views of life-sustaining treatments. Am J Publ Health. 1993;83:14-23.
6. **The SUPPORT Principal Investigators.** A controlled trial to improve care for seriously ill hospitalized patients: the study to understand prognoses and preferences for outcomes and the risk of treatment (SUPPORT). JAMA. 1995; 274:1591-8.
7. **Lee DKP, Swinburne AJ, Fedullo AJ, Wahl GW.** Withdrawing care: experience in a medical intensive care unit. JAMA. 1994;271:1358-61.
8. **Knaus, WA, Wagner DP, Draper EA, et al.** The APACHE III prognostic risk system. Risk prediction of hospital mortality for critically ill hospitalized adults. Chest. 1991;100:1619-36.
9. **Tores D, Lemeshow S, Avrunin SJ, Pastides H.** Validation of the mortality prediction model for ICU patients. Crit Care Med. 1987;15:208-13.
10. **Thibault GE.** Prognosis and clinical predictive models for critically ill patients. In Field MJ, Cassel CK, eds. Approaching Death: Improving Care at the End of Life. Washington, DC: National Academy Press; 1997:363-82.
11. **Rubenfeld G, Crawford S.** Withdrawing life support from mechanically ventilated recipients of bone marrow transplants: a case for evidence-based guidelines. Ann Intern Med. 1996;125:625-33.
12. **Lynn J, Harrell F, Cohn F, et al.** Prognoses of seriously ill hospitalized patients on the days before death: implications for patients care and public policy. New Horiz. 1997;5:56-61.
13. **American Medical Association.** Decisions near the end of life. JAMA. 1992;267:2229-33.
14. **American Thoracic Society.** Withholding and withdrawing life-sustaining therapy. Ann Intern Med. 1991;115;478-84.

15. **Lynn J, Teno JM, Phillips RS, et al.** Perceptions by family members of the dying experience of older and seriously ill patients. Ann Intern Med. 1997;126:97-106.

16. **Hammes BJ, Rooney BL.** Death and end-of-life planning in one Midwestern community. Arch Intern Med. 1998;158:383-90.

17. **Teno JM, Licks, S, Lynn J, et al.** Do advance directives provide instructions that direct care? J Am Geriatr Soc. 1997;45:508-512.

18. **Prendergast TJ.** Resolving conflicts surrounding end-of-life care. New Horiz. 1997;5:62-71.

19. **Caralis PV, Davis B, Wright K, Marcial E.** The influence of ethnicity and race on attitudes toward advance directives, life-prolonging treatments, and euthanasia. J Clin Ethics. 1993;4:155-65.

20. **Leggat JE, Bloembergen WE, Levine G, et al.** An analysis of risk factors for withdrawal from dialysis before death. J Am Soc Nephrol. 1997;8:1755-63

21. **Blackhall, LJ, Murphy ST, Frank G, et al.** Ethnicity and attitudes toward patient autonomy. JAMA. 1995; 274:820-5.

22. **Garrett JM, Harris RP, Norburn JK, et al.** Life-sustaining treatments during terminal illness: who wants what? J Gen Intern Med. 1993;8:361-8.

23. **Haas JS, Weissman JS, Cleary PD, et al.** Discussion of preferences for life-sustaining care by persons with AIDS: predictors of failure in patient-physician communication Arch Intern Med. 1993;153:1241-8.

24. **Koenig, BA.** Cultural diversity in decision making about care at the end of life. In Field MJ, Cassel CK, eds. Approaching Death: Improving Care at the End of Life. Washington, DC: National Academy Press; 1997:363-82.

25. **Faber-Langendoen K, Spomer A, Ingbar D.** A prospective study of withdrawing mechanical ventilation from dying patients. Am J Resp Crit Care Med. 1996;153:4S.

26. **Grenvik A.** "Terminal weaning": discontinuance of life-support therapy in the terminally ill patient. Crit Care Med. 1983;11:394-5.

27. **Prendergast TJ, Luce JM.** Increasing incidence of withholding and withdrawal of life support from the critically ill. Am J Respir Crit Care Med. 1997;155:15-20

28. **Koch KA, Rodeffer HD, Wears RL.** Changing patterns of terminal care management in an intensive care unit. Crit Care Med. 1994;22:233-43.

29. **Christakis N, Asch DA.** Medical specialists prefer to withdraw familiar technologies when discontinuing life support. J Gen Intern Med. 1995;10:491-4.

30. **Christakis N, Asch DA.** Biases in how physicians choose to withdraw life support. Lancet. 1993;342:642-6.

31. **American College of Physicians.** Ethics Manual, 4th ed. Ann Intern Med. 1998:128:576-94.

32. **Lynn J, Childress J.** Must patients always be given food and water? Hastings Center Rep. 1983;13:17-21.

33. **Lo B, Steenbok R.** Beyond the Cruzan case: the U.S. Supreme Court and medical practice. Ann Intern Med. 1991;114:895-901.

34. **King P.** The authority of families to make medical decisions for incompetent patients after the Cruzan decision. Law Med Health Care. 1991:19:76-9.
35. **Miles S.** Futile feeding at the end of life: family virtues and treatment decisions. Theor Med. 1987;8:293-302.
36. **Hamel MB, Phillips RS, Davis RB, et al.** Outcomes and cost-effectiveness of initiating dialysis and continuing aggressive care in seriously ill hospitalized adults. Ann Intern Med. 1997;127:195-202.
37. **Cohen LM, McCue JD, Germain M, Kjellstrand CM.** Dialysis discontinuation: a "good" death? Arch Intern Med. 1995;155:42-7.
38. **Doyle E, Hanks GWC, MacDonald N, eds.** Oxford Textbook of Palliative Medicine. New York: Oxford University Press, 1993;297-89,390-1.
39. **Faber-Langendoen K.** The clinical management of dying patients receiving mechanical ventilation: a survey of physician practice. Chest. 1994;106:880-8.
40. **Gianakos D.** Terminal weaning. Chest. 1995;108:1405-6.
41. **Campbell ML, Frank RR.** Experience with an end-of-life practice at a university hospital. Crit Care Med. 1997;25:197-202.
42. **Gilligan T, Raffin TA.** Withdrawing life support: extubation and prolonged terminal weans are inappropriate. Crit Care Med. 1996; 24:352-3.
43. **Luce JM, Fink C.** Communicating with families about withholding and withdrawal of life support. Chest. 1992;101:1185-6.
44. **Carlson RW, Campbell ML, Frank RR.** Life support: the debate continues. Chest. 1996;109:852-3.
45. **Brody H, Campbell ML, Faber-Langendoen K, Ogle KS.** Withdrawing intensive life-sustaining treatment: recommendations for compassionate clinical management. N Engl J Med. 1997:336:652-7.
46. **Truog RD, Burns JP.** To breathe or not to breathe. J Clin Ethics. 1994;5:39-41.
47. **Quill TE, Barold SS, Sussman BL.** Discontinuing an implantable cardioverter defibrillator as a life-sustaining treatment. Am J Cardiol. 1994;74:205-7.
48. **Spike J.** Retiring the pacemaker. Hastings Center Rep. 1997;27:25-6.
49. **Miller FG, Fins JJ.** A proposal to restructure hospital care for dying patients. N Engl J Med. 1996;334:1740-2.
50. **Pritchard RS, Fisher ES, Teno JM, et al.** Influence of patient preferences and local health system characteristics on the place of death. SUPPORT Invesigators. J Am Geriatr Soc. 1998;46:1242-50.
51. **Byock I.** Dying Well: The Prospect for Growth at the End of Life. New York: Riverhead Books; 1997.

CHAPTER 9

Responding to Intractable Suffering: The Role of Terminal Sedation and Voluntary Refusal of Food and Fluids

TIMOTHY E. QUILL, MD • IRA R. BYOCK, MD

Palliative care that addresses the multiple physical, psychosocial, and spiritual dimensions of suffering should be the standard of care for the dying (1-5). There remain, however, a few patients whose suffering becomes intractable despite excellent care (6-10). This chapter discusses terminal sedation and voluntary refusal of hydration and nutrition as potential last-resort responses to end-of-life suffering that has not otherwise been relieved.

Clinicians who care for severely ill patients must develop expertise in standard palliative care, and they must have strategies for responding to those few patients who face exceptional circumstances. The practices discussed in this paper are, for hospice, palliative care, and geriatric clinicians who oppose physician-assisted suicide, morally and legally preferable responses to severe terminal suffering. The responses to severe terminal suffering presented here may also be acceptable to patients and families who, for reasons of religion or individual values, would not consider suicide or euthanasia.

CASE 9-1. A 66-YEAR-OLD RETIRED RADIOLOGIST WITH GLIOBLASTOMA

BG is a 66-year-old retired radiologist who developed increasing right-sided weakness during several months. CAT scan showed a large, irregular mass deep in the left parietal lobe suggestive of a glioblastoma. After extensive discussions, BG declined biopsy, surgery, radiation therapy, and chemotherapy, electing instead to pursue a purely symptom-oriented approach.

BG is married with two grown children. He was a proud, independent person who valued his intellectual abilities and physical integrity. Although he had not attended church in recent years, he was a life-long Unitarian and had a long history of involvement in progressive social issues. In his work as a radiologist, he had seen the downward course of many patients with brain tumors and wanted no part of it. He understood that there could be limited success with treatment, but he was unwilling to subject himself and his family to the significant burdens it would entail. He did not want to die but was fearful of becoming physically dependent on his family and of being intellectually impaired and unable to make his own decisions. He had a series of long talks with his family, his primary physician, and several specialists before finally making up his mind.

The initial goal of the palliative plan of care was to manage his symptoms so that he could have as much quality time with his wife and children as possible. Corticosteroids and antiseizure medications were the central symptom-relieving measures. His symptoms improved for several weeks as he and his family worked to achieve closure in their lives together. They reviewed the family photo album and shared stories. BG achieved a closeness with his family that he had often missed during his years of long work hours as a physician. His hospice nurse also visited him regularly, as did his Unitarian minister.

Unfortunately, BG's right-sided weakness began to rapidly worsen, and he developed focal motor seizures despite antiepileptic medication, which left him weakened and slightly disoriented for several hours after each episode. Sensing his physical and intellectual deterioration, BG wanted to get on with it before, "I can't do anything for myself." When asked what he meant, fear of further mental and physical deterioration were more disturbing to him than the prospect of death. He had no moral qualms about hastening his death, although he did not want to compromise his physician or his family by requesting medicine for an overdose. He hoped he could die by stopping his dexamethasone, and he knew he had a legal right to refuse unwanted treatment. A consulting psychiatrist confirmed that BG understood his treatment options and was not clinically depressed. After saying goodbyes to friends and family, BG discontinued his dexamethasone, hoping that he would slip into a coma and die. He was reassured that any significant headache could be treated with opioid analgesics.

To BG's consternation, he did not become comatose or die. Instead, his right-sided weakness worsened, and his seizures became more frequent. Although he experienced only mild headaches, which responded to acetaminophen and hydrocodone, he requested morphine to relieve his suffering. BG found his situation intolerable and became desperate to "get it over with one way or another." He did not explicitly request medication that could be taken in a lethal overdose, but his desire for a hastened death was clear. "I just want to go to sleep and not wake up," he said on several occasions.

BG's physicians, the hospice team, and his minister were committed to relieving his distress. Together, they tried to improve his seizure management and his mood while enhancing family support during this challenging time. An empiric trial of methylphenidate lightened his mood slightly but did not change his resolve to not continue living under his current circumstances. His physician wondered if terminal sedation and voluntarily refusal of food and fluids could be options for BG, but she was unsure what each involved or how they should be discussed.

The Clinical Problem

Comprehensive palliative care is effective for most dying patients (11-17), but there remain a few people whose suffering becomes extreme and intolerable in spite of skillful, maximal efforts (6-10). Survey data show that 5% to 35% of patients in hospice programs report their pain as being "severe" in the last week of life and 25% report their shortness of breath as "unbearable" (8). On occasion, physical symptoms such as terminal delirium, severe bleeding, weakness, open wounds, profound weight loss, and seizures challenge even the most experienced hospice teams.

Data from the Netherlands and the United States suggest that requests for physician-assisted death infrequently come from unrelieved pain alone. They more commonly result from a combination of physical symptoms and debility, weakness, lack of meaning, and tiredness of living under the circumstances imposed by the illness (18-21). The relevant suffering of the terminally ill is, therefore, a complex amalgam of pain, physical symptoms, and psychosocial, existential, and spiritual suffering, as balanced by hope, love, connection, and meaning (22-26). Understanding each patient's unique suffering, and responding to it in a multi-faceted way, is at the crux of palliative medicine. Suffering may arise from a sense of impending disintegration of one's person (22) or from an experienced loss of meaning (23) that may have little to do with uncontrolled physical symptoms.

BG's suffering was not simple to categorize. His progressive inability to participate in life in ways he found meaningful was at its core. He feared being a burden to his family and progressive loss of mental capacity more than uncontrolled pain. In this sense, his suffering was a combination of psychological, existential, and physical factors. For BG's physician, understanding her patient's core values clarified the nature of his distress, and helped identify potential approaches to its relief. Furthermore, BG had no particular moral reservations about hastening death in the setting of severe suffering. For him, the humaneness and effectiveness of the intervention were more important than whether it required "active" or "passive" assistance by his physician.

A primary clinical concern when a patient requests a hastened death, whether by forgoing life-extending treatment, stopping eating and drinking, or by terminal sedation, is the assessment of decision-making capacity (27-31). Potentially treatable affective disorders are common but not well recognized in the terminally ill (27-30). In one small study of hospice patients, 60% of those requesting assisted suicide met criteria for clinical depression, but the remaining 40% had no definable mental disorder (32). Because the symptoms of terminal illness overlap considerably with depression, diagnosis can be challenging, and criteria may need to be modified in order to focus on distortion of judgment, hopelessness out of proportion to the situation, and capacity for informed consent (27-30,32-36). If there is doubt about the patient's decision-making capacity, formal assessment by a mental health professional should be undertaken. BG's primary physician prevailed upon him to be evaluated by a psychiatrist before lending her support to his decision to stop dexamethasone.

Terminal Sedation

The use of high doses of analgesics and/or sedatives to relieve extremes of physical distress is not restricted to end-of-life care. It is sometimes employed as a temporizing measure in trauma, burn, post-surgical, and intensive care; although rendering a patient unconscious is an unusual intervention, in circumstances such as these it seems inhumane to not do so. Careful attention is paid to maintaining adequate ventilation, hydration, and nutrition because these patients are expected to recover from the traumatic event.

Terminal sedation, on the other hand, refers to a similar response to the extremes of physical suffering in patients who are imminently dying (7,37-41). The medications are always justified by the obligation to avoid suffering, and not to purposefully end the patient's life (42). However, unlike the situation in which recovery is expected, other life-prolonging interventions such as mechanical ventilation and artificial hydration are avoided because they are considered to be inconsistent with the patient's goals of care. In the context of end-of-life care, the component practices of intensive symptom management and withholding of life-sustaining treatment have widespread ethical and legal support (31,43-46). However, because death is a foreseeable and inevitable outcome of the aggregated circumstances of the patient's condition and interventions, the act has the potential for more moral complexity and ambiguity than is often acknowledged (31,45,47). Therefore, terminal sedation has been inconsistently available at the end of life.

Terminal sedation should be distinguished from the much more common situation of a dying patient gradually slipping into an obtunded state as death approaches, an indirect and unintended consequence of the metabolic changes of dying in combination with usual palliative treatments. Rather, terminal sedation involves an explicit decision to render the patient unconscious to prevent otherwise unrelievable suffering. Although the medical purpose of treatment is to relieve intolerable suffering, it is acknowledged that death may be preferred by the patient to his or her current situation. When a patient or physician views terminal sedation as a means for hastening death, its moral status may become more complex (31,45). Nonetheless, there is growing acceptance of the practice when used as a last resort with the intention of responding to severe, otherwise unrelievable suffering. Indeed, in circumstances in which a dying patient's physical suffering is profound and in which other interventions are unavailable or have previously failed, the failure to offer sedation may represent a form of patient abandonment (48).

Voluntary Refusal of Food and Fluids

In this situation, a competent patient makes the conscious choice to stop the oral intake of food and fluid even though he or she is still physically capable of eating and drinking (49-52). When voluntary stopping eating and drinking results from an active patient choice with the intention of hastening death, the practice is usually distinguishable from the "natural" anorexia and loss of thirst that frequently accompany the very end stages of dying, although in some cases the processes may overlap. A patient's decision to stop eating and drinking can be categorized ethically as a decision to forgo life-sustaining therapies (49-52). However, some consider it to be a form of suicide because the patient is explicitly and voluntarily hastening death (31). The patient's decision to refuse food and fluids is neither physician-ordered nor directed, yet in practice it requires the support of the family and the health care team to provide usual palliative treatment and support as the dying process unfolds (53).

During food and fluid fasts, any uncomfortable symptoms that emerge will need palliation. In the context of advanced oncologic illnesses, hunger is rare and transient, and symptoms of dry mouth and throat usually respond to assiduous mouth care (54). Dying under these circumstances can take several days to a few weeks, depending on the patient's disease burden and nutritional and metabolic state at the outset. Doubts on the part of the family or physician may arise as the process unfolds, especially if the process is prolonged or if the patient develops pre-terminal delirium. If a specific food or drink is transiently requested, whether or not it occurs in the context of confusion, we believe it is reasonable to offer it on a one-time basis. If such requests persist, the decision and therapeutic response demand re-evaluation involving the patient and family. The health care team can help the family confront these challenging questions, maintaining focus on the patient's wishes and comfort, while being open to the possibility that the patient is choosing a different course. If a patient becomes severely agitated in the process of stopping eating and drinking as death approaches, intensive symptom management, even including terminal sedation, is indicated as required to provide comfort.

Moral and Legal Status

Although public discussion about terminal sedation and stopping eating and drinking is less developed compared to other end-of-life decisions, the June 1997 United States Supreme Court decision on assisted suicide strongly suggested that they are permitted under current law (46,55,56). The Court unequivocally supported the right to refuse treatment, even if the patient's intention is to hasten death, based on the patient's interest in bodily integrity. Furthermore, Justice Souter's concurrence supported the practice of terminal sedation: "The State permits physicians to administer medication to patients in terminal conditions where the primary intent is to relieve pain, even when the medication is so powerful as to hasten death and the patient chooses to receive it with that understanding" (55,56).

Public and professional discussion of the moral status of these practices is now underway (31,42-46,52,57). In Supreme Court briefs opposing physician-assisted suicide, terminal sedation and stopping eating and drinking were presented by hospice, palliative care, and geriatrics groups as morally acceptable responses of last resort when suffering cannot otherwise be satisfactorily relieved, and the patient consents (58,59). The Supreme Court briefs presented these practices as currently available and more morally acceptable than physician-assisted suicide because death is not directly or intentionally hastened by the physician. In addition, terminal sedation and patient refusal to eat and drink can respond to a much wider range of suffering and clinical circumstances than physician-assisted suicide, even if the latter were legalized. They do not require the patient's ability to ingest medications or take other life-ending actions independently, and support can be provided and monitored within usual health care settings.

Moral Questions

Are These Practices Fundamentally Different from Physician-Assisted Suicide?

An in-depth comparison of these options of last resort has been presented elsewhere (31,52,57-59). For many clinicians and patients, the differences between terminal sedation and voluntarily stopping eating and drinking on the one hand and physician-assisted suicide and voluntary euthanasia on the other are fundamental (44,52,57), and for others they are all more similar than different (42,43,45). Many clinicians who believe that the physician should never knowingly and intentionally hasten death find their role in supporting terminal sedation or voluntarily stopping eating and drinking to be entirely consistent with their obligation to palliate symptoms and suffering (44,52,57). Many of these practitioners cannot support physician-assisted suicide, but these options give them a morally acceptable way to respond to severe terminal suffering without abandoning the patient and family. Similarly, many patients and their families who could never support "suicide" find these practices an acceptable last resort option. As an example, one religious patient suffering severely on a home hospice program viewed her voluntary cessation of eating and drinking as a "fast for God."

When a Patient Seeks These Interventions as a Means for Hastening Death, Does That Make the Practices Tantamount to Suicide?

For many clinicians and bioethicists, the moral evaluation of these practices depends in part on their clinical context. For a patient with anorexia nervosa, clinical depression, or mildly symptomatic illness, stopping eating and drinking would be considered a form of suicide to be prevented by appropriate interventions. In contrast, for a patient with severe, unrelieved suffering and a progressive, incurable illness, the same acts might be supported within the right to refuse treatment (31,52,57). Some clinicians and ethicists, however, believe that any and all intentional hastening of death by a patient would constitute suicide, and they consider any physician involvement to be unacceptable. The absolute prohibition of physician participation creates a double bind for patients who are ready for death and desire the help of their physician. If such patients are honest about their desire and intention to hasten death, a request for physician support cannot be granted. If, however, these patients deceive their care providers by not disclosing their desires and, instead, present their request for help as a need for more intensive symptom management, the assistance of a physician can be permitted. Ethics, clinical protocols, and physician practice should encourage patients to be honest and forthright about their feelings, desires, and intentions. Professional caregivers should be as responsive to the stated needs and preferences of patients as possible, without violating their own fundamental values.

Are Physicians Required to Support Requests for These Practices?

It is incumbent on physicians who care for severely ill patients to fully explore patient requests for terminal sedation or voluntarily stopping eating and drinking, and to ensure that these requests are not emanating from unrecognized depression or symptoms that may respond to palliative measures. Physicians would not be required, however, to provide either of these interventions if it violated fundamental personal moral precepts (31). If physicians cannot find common ground with such a patient, they have a responsibility to obtain palliative care and/or ethics consultations. Because sedation for refractory symptoms and refusal to eat and drink in these circumstances have legal support and because they have been endorsed by many within the palliative care, ethics, and geriatrics communities, patients should be given the option of transferring care to a more receptive physician if possible.

Additional Questions

How frequently will terminal sedation and refusal of food and drink be employed in the presence of state-of-the-art palliative care? How acceptable will either of these options be to patients, families, and health care providers? Will predictable availability of these options of last resort diminish patient fears about physician abandonment in the face of severe end-of-life suffering? Will these options lessen public interest in assisted suicide? Will discussion of these options make some patients more fearful about physician power and potential abuse? If care of this nature was predictably available, how many patients would still prefer assisted suicide, and how many physicians would still covertly break the law by providing assistance? Do patients, families, and physicians see these actions as morally different from physician-assisted suicide or euthanasia? If voluntary refusal of food and fluids is considered a type of forgoing life-sustaining measure, should it be available to incurably ill and suffering patients who are not imminently terminal?

Clinical Guidelines and Practicalities

The published guidelines in the palliative care literature for terminal sedation and voluntarily stopping eating and drinking have similarities and differences (31,38). Informed consent is the first cornerstone, and it includes assessing the patient's capacity to comprehend the treatment and the available alternatives. A careful evaluation of confounding depression or evidence of cognitive distortion must be undertaken, with involvement of a mental health professional if there is uncertainty (60,61). Whereas full decision-making capacity is an absolute requirement for voluntarily stopping eating and drinking, terminal sedation may sometimes be needed for acute symptomatic emergencies when the dying patient cannot respond and surrogates are not available. In such severe circumstances, the patient's values may have to be represented by consultants or other members of the health care team.

The second cornerstone is the presence of severe suffering that cannot be relieved by other available means. The main indication for terminal sedation has been severe physical suffering such as intractable pain, dyspnea, or seizures, uncontrolled by ordinary means. Refusal of food and fluids may be considered by patients who have more unrelenting, persistent symptoms that are unacceptable, such as extreme fatigue, weakness, or debility.

If terminal sedation or refusal of food and fluids is being considered by a patient who is not imminently dying, assessments should always include second opinions from mental health and palliative care specialists. Substantial waiting periods and clinical trials of psychopharmacologic measures should be considered if there is substantial uncertainty about the patient's mental capacity or the intractability of suffering. Table 9-1 summarizes the general guidelines for terminal sedation and voluntary refusal of food and fluids. Terminal sedation and stopping of food and fluids should be employed with caution and only in the most difficult cases. Situations of this nature are typically marked by struggle on the part of the physician, the clinical team, the family, and the patient. This struggle is unavoidable and necessary, a mark of caring intention and authenticity that contributes to the moral acceptability of the choices made. Ethics, palliative care, and/or psychiatric consultations should be obtained on cases where substantial uncertainty remains.

Terminal sedation can be achieved with a barbiturate or benzodiazepine infusion, rapidly increased until the patient is adequately sedated and appears free from discomfort. A level of sedation sufficient to obviate signs of discomfort (such as stiffening or grimacing spontaneously or with routine repositioning and nursing care) is maintained until the patient dies. Table 9-2 shows potential starting doses and strategies for increasing doses and monitoring. In some special circumstances, with the patient's previous consent, sedation can periodically be lightened to evaluate the patient's subjective experience and confirm his or her preferences for care. Depending on the severity of the patient's physiologic condition at the onset, the time interval from initiation to death can be hours to days, to occasionally even a week or more. Terminal sedation requires intensive monitoring and observation by the health care team. When a dying patient requires sedation, opioids for pain and other symptom-relieving measures should be continued to avoid the possibility of unobservable pain or opioid withdrawal. Because tolerance develops to the sedating effects of opioids, doses may need to be increased over time to achieve continuous sedation if the opiods are not combined with sedatives.

Evaluating a patient who is considering voluntarily stopping eating and drinking similarly requires a careful assessment of mental status, an investigation of why suffering has become so intolerable at this

Table 9-1. General Guidelines for Terminal Sedation and Voluntary Refusal of Food and Fluids.

Guideline Domain	Terminal Sedation	Voluntary Refusal of Food and Fluids
Palliative care	Must be available, in place, and unable to relieve current suffering adequately	Must be available, in place, and unable to relieve current suffering adequately
Usual patient characteristics	Severe, immediate, otherwise unrelievable symptoms (e.g., pain, shortness of breath, nausea, vomiting, seizures, delirium); terminal sedation can be used to prevent severe suffering (e.g., to prevent suffocation sensation when discontinuing mechanical ventilation)	Persistent, unrelenting, otherwise unrelievable symptoms unacceptable to the patient (e.g., extreme fatigue, weakness, debility)
Terminal prognosis	Usually days to weeks	Usually weeks to months
Patient informed consent	Patient competent, fully informed; or incompetent with severe, otherwise irreversible suffering (use advance directive and/or consensus about patient wishes and best interests)	Patient competent, fully informed
Family participation in decision	Strongly encourage input from and consensus of immediate family members	Strongly encourage input from and consensus of immediate family members
Incompetent patient	Terminal sedation available for indications of severe persistent suffering with the informed consent of the patient's designated proxy, family members; if no surrogate available, consensus from team members and consultants that no other acceptable palliative responses are available	Food and drink (oral food and fluids) must not be withheld from incompetent persons willing and able to eat
Second opinion(s)	Expert in palliative care; mental health expert (if uncertainty about mental capacity)	Expert in palliative care; mental health expert; specialist in the patient's underlying disease (strongly advised)
Medical staff participation in decision	Input from staff involved in immediate patient care activities encouraged; physician and staff consent for their own participation required	Input from staff involved in immediate patient care activities encouraged; physician and staff consent for their own participation required

Table 9-2.   Medications Used for Terminal Sedation.

Medication	Type	Usual Starting Dose	Usual Maintenance Dose	Route
Midazolam	Rapid and short acting benzodi-azepine	0.5-1.5 mg/hr after bolus of 0.5 mg	30-100 mg/day	Intravenous or subcutaneous
Lorazepam	Benzodi-azepine	1-4 mg q 4-6 h po or dissolved buccally; infusion of 0.5-1.0 mg/hr intravenously	4-40 mg/day	Orally, buccally subcutaneous-ly, or intra-venously
Propofol	General anesthetic; ultra-rapid onset and elimination	5-10 mg/hr, bolus doses of 20-50 mg may be administered for urgent sedation but continuous infu-sion required	10-200 mg/hr	Intravenous
Thiopental	Ultra-short acting barbiturate	5-7 mg/kg to induce unconsciousness	Initial rate may range from 20-80 mg/hr; average main-tenance rates range from 70-180 mg/hr	Intravenous
Pentobarbital	Long-acting barbiturate	2-3 mg/kg slow infu-sion to induce unconsciousness	1 mg/hr, increasing as needed to maintain sedation	Intravenous
Phenobarbital	Long-acting barbiturate	200 mg loading dose, repeated q 10-15 min until patient is comfortable	About 50 mg/hr	Intravenous or subcutaneous

1. Goal of treatment is to relieve suffering by inducing sedation.
2. Dose should be increased by about 30% every hour until sedation is achieved.
3. Once desired level of sedation is achieved, infusion is usually maintained at that level as long as patient appears comfortable.
4. If symptoms return, doses should be increased in 30% increments until sedation is achieved.
5. The dose ranges above are representative. Individual patients may require lower or higher doses to achieve the desired goal.
6. Prior doses of opioids and other symptom-relieving medications should be continued.

Table Bibliography
Cherny NI, Portenoy RK. Sedation in the management of refractory symptoms. J Palliat Care. 1994;10:31-8.
Dunlop RJ. Is terminal restlessness sometimes drug induced? Palliative Med. 1989;3 (1):65-6.
Enck RE. The Medical Care of Terminally Ill Patients. Baltimore: Johns Hopkins University Press. 1994:166-72.
Greene WR, Davis WH. Titrated Intravenous barbiturates in the control of symptoms in patients with ter-minal cancer. So Med J. 1991;84:332-7.
Hanks GWC, MacDonald N, Doyle D. eds. Oxford Textbook of Palliative Medicine. Oxford University Press. 1998:945-7.
Moyle, J. The use of propofol in palliative medicine. J Pain Symptom Manage. 1995;10:643-6.
Truog RD, Berde CB, Mitchell C, Grier HE. Barbiturates in the care of the terminally ill. N Eng J Med. 1992;327:1678-82.

point in time, and a wide-ranging search for less drastic palliative care alternatives. Although the patient's refusal of food and fluids technically does not require the physician's participation, a physician should be part of the team who will assess the patient's request, and then provide palliative care to the patient and family as the process unfolds. On occasion, particularly if agitated delirium develops as the patient dehydrates, intensive palliative measures including terminal sedation may subsequently be needed. Therefore, a physician who opposes the patient's decision from the outset must decide whether or not he or she can provide all forms of palliation that may be indicated. If the physician feels morally unable to do so, transfer of care to another provider should be attempted.

Discussing these options of last resort with all patients with late-stage illness would seem burdensome and inappropriate to both patients and physicians. All severely ill patients with substantial suffering and poor prognosis should be informed about the potential of palliative care to address their symptoms and suffering. In contrast, information about terminal sedation and stopping eating and drinking becomes appropriate when patients express fears about dying badly or explicitly request a hastened death because of unacceptable suffering. Terminal sedation may also be considered preventively for dying patients who are discontinuing life-sustaining therapy such as mechanical ventilation yet fear suffocation. For patients who fear dying badly, discussion of these possibilities can provide reassurance that their physicians will effectively respond to their suffering and avoid prolonging conditions the patients view as "worse than death." This knowledge may allow some people to avoid worrying about future physical agony and to focus more energy on matters of life closure and completion. The information must be presented with considerable sensitivity, however, because people might experience being offered these options as subtle coercion, imposing a burden by requiring them to justify their decision to keep living. Still others might find the prospect of spending their final days in an iatrogenic coma to be meaningless and undignified and prefer a more decisive action such as assisted suicide.

Medicine cannot sanitize dying, nor can it provide perfect solutions for all clinical dilemmas. Nonetheless, offering terminal sedation or voluntary stopping eating and drinking to selected patients who suffer severely and request a hastened death extends the range of options that can be openly considered and medically supported during this inherently difficult time in human life. Patients who fear that physicians will not respond to extremes of suffering will be reassured when such options are reliably available. Relevant professional bodies can help by adopting policy statements attesting to the ethical and professional acceptability of these aspects of palliative care.

In response to BG's repeated comments about wanting to "get this over with," his physician raised the possibility of stopping eating and drinking and promised to use medications to induce a "twilight sleep" sedation if his suffering became intolerable in the process of dying. BG said he had never considered "starving myself" because he assumed it would add to his suffering. He reflected that he hadn't been hungry for many weeks and said he felt liberated by being made aware of a choice he could pursue openly, by his own volition. The prospect of a two-week period before death after the decision to stop food and fluids was not an excessive burden in BG's view. It would allow him some time to again say goodbye to his family, but with a predictable beginning, middle, and end. Both he and his family were reassured that any additional symptoms that emerged would be aggressively managed. BG and his physician each spoke with the consulting neurologist and psychiatrist. BG also discussed his decision at length with his wife, children, and minister.

Two days later, BG stopped eating and drinking. The initial week was physically comfortable and personally meaningful. BG's family shared stories, played cards, and listened to music. BG took antiseizure medications and methylphenidate with sips of water, but absolutely nothing else orally. Morphine by continuous subcutaneous infusion at an initial dose of 1.0 mg/hr controlled his headaches without causing sedation. His mouth was kept moist with ice chips and swabs, but he was careful not to swallow any of the liquid. He denied feeling hunger, and had no significant discomfort from thirst other than occasional dry mouth. He began spending much of the day and night sleeping and after 9 days was too weak to swallow his medications. He then began to have hallucinations, some of which appeared to be terrifying. The peace and comfort that had been achieved for BG and his family began to unravel.

BG was now incapable of informed consent but had pre-viously given permission for sedation if this type of problem arose. After discussions with his family, BG was started on a low-dose subcutaneous infusion of midazolam for treatment of seizures and agitation. The initial dose was 0.5 mg/hr with bolus doses of 0.5 to 1 mg ordered up to every 15 min as need-ed. The option of transferring BG to an inpatient unit was explored, but the family preferred to keep him at home. Twenty-four hour home nursing care was arranged under the continuous care provision of the Medicare Hospice Benefit. After several bolus doses and adjustment of the infusion to 2.5 mg/hr over the first 6 hours, BG appeared to be sleeping com-fortably. No further increases in medication were needed. BG died quietly approximately 24 hours later in his home, with a hospice nurse in attendance and his entire family surround-ing his bed. The family struggled at times as to whether they were doing too little or too much to help him die peacefully, but generally felt that they had kept BG's values at the forefront and made the best of a potentially devastating situation.

REFERENCES

1. **ABIM End-of-Life Patient Care Project Committee.** Caring for the Dying: Identification and Promotion of Physician Competence. Educational resource document. Philadelphia: ABIM; 1996.
2. **American Medical Association, Council on Ethical and Judicial Affairs.** Decisions near the end of life. JAMA. 1992;276:2229-33.
3. **American Medical Association, Council on Scientific Affairs.** Good care for the dying patient. JAMA. 1996;275:474-8.
4. **Field MJ, Cassel CK, eds., for the Institute of Medicine, Committee on Care at the End of Life.** Approaching Death: Improving Care at the End of Life. Washington, DC: National Academy Press; 1997.
5. **Meier DM, Block SD, Billings JA.** The debate over physician-assisted sui-cide: empirical data and convergent views. Ann Intern Med. 1998;128:552-8.
6. **Kasting GA.** The nonnecessity of euthanasia. In: Humber JD, Almeder RJ, Kasting GA, eds. Physician-Assisted Death. Totawa, New Jersey: Humana Press; 1993:25-43.
7. **Ventafrida V, Ripamonti C, DeConno F, Tamburini M.** Symptom preva-lence and control during cancer patient's last days of life. J Palliat Care. 1990;6:7-11.
8. **Coyle N, Adelhardt J, Foley KM, Portenoy RK.** Character of terminal illness in the advanced cancer patient: pain and other symptoms during the last four weeks of life. J Pain Symptom Manage. 1990;5:83-93.

9. **Ingham J, Portenoy R.** Symptom assessment. Hematol Oncol Clin North Am. 1996:10:21-39.

10. **Quill TE, Brody RV.** "You promised me I wouldn't die like this": a bad death as a medical emergency. Arch Intern Med. 1995;155:1250?4.

11. **Seale CF.** What happens in hospices: a review of research evidence. Soc Sci Med. 1989;28:551-9.

12. **Wallston KA, Burger C, Smith RA, Baugher RJ.** Comparing the quality of death for hospice and non-hospice cancer patients. Med Care. 1998;26:177-82.

13. **Byock I.** Dying Well: Prospects for Growth at the End of Life. New York: Riverhead Books; 1997.

14. **Foley KM.** Pain, physician-assisted suicide and euthanasia. Pain Forum. 1995;4:163-78.

15. **Hadad AR, Browman GP.** The WHO analgesic ladder for cancer pain management: stepping up the quality of its evaluation. JAMA. 1995;274:1870-3.

16. **American Pain Society Quality of Care Committee.** Quality improvement guidelines for the treatment of acute pain and cancer pain. JAMA. 1995;274:1874-80.

17. **Rhymes J.** Hospice in America. JAMA. 1990;264:369-72.

18. **Back AL, Wallace JI, Starks HE, Pearlman RA.** Physician-assisted suicide and euthanasia in Washington State: patient requests and physician responses. JAMA. 1996;275:919-25.

19. **van der Maas PJ, van Delden JJM, Pijnenborg L.** Euthanasia and other medical decisions concerning the end of life. Health Policy, vol 2. Amsterdam: Elsevier; 1992.

20. **Meier D, Emmons C. Wallenstein S, et al.** A national survey of physician-assisted suicide and euthanasia in the United States. N Engl J Med. 1998;338:1193-201.

21. **vanderMaas PJ, vanderWal, G, Haverkate I, et al.** Euthanasia, physician-assisted suicide, and other medical practices involving the end of life in the Netherlands, 1990-1995. N Engl J Med. 1996;335:1699-1705.

22. **Cassell EJ.** The nature of suffering and the goals of medicine. N Engl J Med. 1992;306:639-45.

23. **Frankel VE.** The Doctor and the Soul. New York: Vintage Books; 1955.

24. **Byock I.** The nature of suffering and the nature of opportunity at the end of life. Clin Geriatr Med. 1996;12:237-51.

25. **Byock I.** When suffering persists. J Palliat Care. 1994;10:8-13.

26. **Quill TE.** A Midwife Through the Dying Process: Stories of Healing and Hard Choices at the End of Life. Baltimore: Johns Hopkins University Press; 1997.

27. **Kathol RG, Noyes R, Williams J, et al.** Diagnosing depression in patients with medical illness. Psychosomatics. 1990;31:434-40.

28. **Sullivan MD, Youngner SJ.** Depression, competence and the right to refuse lifesaving medical treatment. Am J Psychiatry. 1994;151:971-8.

29. **Conwell Y, Caine ED.** Rational suicide and the right to die: reality and myth. N Engl J Med. 1991;325:1100-3.

30. **Chochinov HM, Wilson KG, Enns M, Lander S.** Prevalence of depression in the terminally ill: effects of diagnostic criteria and symptom threshold judgments. Am J Psychiatry. 1994;151:537-40.

31. **Quill TE, Lo B, Brock D.** Palliative options of last resort: a comparison of voluntarily stopping eating and drinking, terminal sedation, physician-assisted suicide and voluntary active euthanasia. JAMA. 1997;278:2099-104.

32. **Chochinov JM, Wilson KG, Enns M, et al.** Desire for death in the terminally ill. Am J Psychiatry. 1995;152:1185-91.

33. **Emanuel EJ, Fairclough DL, Daniels ER, Clarridge BR.** Euthanasia and physician-assisted suicide: attitudes and experiences of oncology patients, oncologists, and the public. Lancet. 1996;347:1805-10.

34. **Breitbart W, Rosenfeld BD, Passik SD.** Interest in physician-assisted suicide among ambulatory HIV-infected patients. Am J Psychiatry. 1996;153:238-42.

35. **Lee MA, Ganzini L.** Depression in the elderly: effect on patient attitudes toward life-sustaining therapy. J Am Geriat Society. 1992;40:983-8.

36. **Ganzini L, Lee MA, Heintz RT, et al.** The effect of depression treatment on elderly patients' preferences for life-sustaining therapy. Am J Psychiatry. 994;151:1631-6.

37. **Troug RD, Berde DB, Mitchell C, Grier HE.** Barbiturates in the care of the terminally ill. N Engl J Med. 1991;327:1678-81.

38. **Cherney NI, Portenoy RK.** Sedation in the management of refractory symptoms: guidelines for evaluation and treatment. J Palliat Care. 1994;10:31-8.

39. **Enck RE.** The Medical Care of Terminally Ill Patients. Baltimore: Johns Hopkins University Press; 1994.

40. **Saunders C, Sykes N.** The Management of Terminal Malignant Disease, 3rd ed. London: Hodder; 1993.

41. **Stone P, Phillips C, Spruyt O, Waight C.** A comparison of the use of sedatives in a hospital support team and in a hospice. Palliat Med. 1997;11:140-4.

42. **Quill TE, Dresser R, Brock DW.** The rule of double effect: a critique of its role in end-of-life decision making. N Engl J Med. 1997;337:1768-71.

43. **Brody H.** Causing, intending, and assisting death. J Clin Ethics. 1993;4:112-7.

44. **Byock IR.** Consciously walking the fine line: thoughts on a hospice response to assisted suicide and euthanasia. J Palliat Care. 1993;9:25?8.

45. **Billings JA, Block S.** Slow euthanasia. J Palliat Care. 1996;12:21-30.

46. **Burt RA.** The Supreme Court speaks: not assisted suicide but a constitutional right to palliative care. N Engl J Med. 1997;337:1234-6.

47. **Quill TE.** The ambiguity of clinical intentions. N Engl J Med. 1993;329:1039-40.

48. **Quill TE, Cassel CK.** Nonabandonment: a central obligation for physicians. Ann Intern Med. 1995;122:368-74.

49. **Bernat JL, Gert B, Mogielnicki RP.** Patient refusal of hydration and nutrition: an alternative to physician-assisted suicide or voluntary active euthanasia? Arch Intern Med. 1993;153:2723-7.

50. **Printz LA.** Terminal dehydration: a compassionate treatment. Arch Intern Med. 1992;152:697-700.

51. **Eddy DM.** A conversation with my mother. JAMA. 1994;272:179-81.
52. **Miller FG, Meier DE.** Voluntary death: a comparison of terminal dehydration and physician-assisted suicide. Ann Intern Med. 1998;128:559-62.
53. **Brody H, Campbell ML, Faber-Langendoen K, Ogle KS.** Withdrawing intensive life-sustaining treatment: recommendations for compassionate clinical management. N Engl J Med. 1997;336:652-7.
54. **McCann RM, Hall WJ, Groth-Juncker A.** Comfort care for terminally ill patients. JAMA. 1994;272:1263-6.
55. Vacco v. Quill, 117 S.Ct. 2293 (1997).
56. Washington v. Glucksberg, 117 S.Ct. 2258 (1997).
57. **Byock I.** Patient refusal of nutrition and hydration: walking the ever-finer line. Am J Hospice Palliat Care. March/April 1995; 8-13.
58. **Lynn J, Cohn F. Pickering JH, et al.** American Geriatrics Society on Physician-Assisted Suicide: Brief to the United States Supreme Court. JAGS. 1997;45:489-99.
59. Brief Amicus Curiae for the National Hospice Organization in Vacco v. Quill and Washington v. Glucksberg, Supreme Court of the United States, Oct. 1996.
60. **Quill TE.** "Doctor, I want to die. Will you help me?" JAMA. 1993;270:870-3.
61. **Block SD, Billings JA.** Patient requests to hasten death: evaluation and management in terminal care. Arch Intern Med. 1994;154:2039-47.

CHAPTER 10

Life After Death: A Practical Approach to Grief and Bereavement

DAVID J. CASARETT, MD, MA • JEAN S. KUTNER, MD •
JANET L. ABRAHM, MD

"The dead want nothing of us but that we live."

Gain—Richard Powers

t some point in their personal and professional lives, all physicians will encounter grief and loss. They will experience the deaths of friends, family members, and patients, but they will also observe the grief that their patients experience. Grief may be overt (the widower who presents with depression soon after the death of his wife), but it may be less obvious (the woman who describes fatigue and insomnia at a routine gynecology examination).

It is important that physicians recognize grief, most importantly because it is distressing to patients, but also because grief may manifest as a variety of somatic complaints and should especially be considered as a possible cause of symptoms that occur near the time of a loved one's death (1,2). Bereaved persons appear to be at increased risk of health problems, suicide, and other causes of death (3), so physicians should be aware of grief as a cause of somatic complaints and as a predictor of illness in the bereaved population.

Despite its importance, however, grief has remained outside the province of medicine (4). This is not to say that physicians have ignored grief entirely. For instance, Benjamin Rush viewed grief as one of the most profound threats to health, and advocated an aggressive course of bleeding and purging for his bereaved patients (5). Even if his approach was dubious, his enthusiasm was admirable.

Nevertheless, this enthusiasm has still not been embraced in mainstream medical practice.

To help physicians include grief as a routine part of care, this chapter presents the experiences of a dying patient, Mr. Powsand, and his wife. First, anticipatory grief, or the grief response that occurs before death, is described. Next, an acute grief reaction (Mrs. Powsand's reaction to her husband's death) is considered. Then the typical features of grief that occur later in the grieving process are detailed. The chapter concludes with a description of grief that has become "complicated."

Throughout this narrative, the physician plays a relatively small part. This is because the vast majority of the support that people receive after a loss comes from friends and family, rather than from physicians. The physician does, however, play an important part in a patient's grieving process. There are clear opportunities for physicians to make a difference in identifying problems and in orchestrating resources.

Anticipatory Grief

CASE 10-1. A 67-YEAR-OLD MAN WITH SEVERE ISCHEMIC CARDIOMYOPATHY AND INOPERABLE CORONARY ARTERY DISEASE

Mr. Powsand is a 67-year-old married man with severe ischemic cardiomyopathy and inoperable coronary artery disease. He has been hospitalized six times during the past year for exacerbations of heart failure and has required admission to the intensive care unit on several occasions. During the past 2 years of his illness, his wife of 29 years has gradually taken over their affairs. Dr. Wedlich is seeing him in a routine office visit. Mrs. Powsand, who has driven him to the office, is in the waiting room. When Dr. Wedlich asks Mr. Powsand how things have been going, the patient says that he thinks he's doing "fair," but that he's worried about his wife. When Dr. Wedlich inquires further, Mr. Powsand says that she seems anxious and that he has seen her crying when she doesn't think he is look-

ing. She has also stopped attending her weekly bridge game. Mr. Powsand asks whether anything can be done to help her.

Given the brief description that Mr. Powsand has provided, it seems likely that Mrs. Powsand is experiencing anticipatory grief. This term describes the process of slowly coming to terms with the potential loss of a significant person. This is a multidimensional syndrome consisting of anger, guilt, anxiety, irritability, sadness, feelings of loss, and decreased ability to function at usual tasks (6) (Table 10-1).

If Mrs. Powsand is experiencing anticipatory grief, Dr. Wedlich has several opportunities to provide support for her (Table 10-2). He should begin by asking to talk to Mr. and Mrs. Powsand together. The goal of this discussion should be to confirm Mr. Powsand's observations and to help the couple talk about the changes in Mrs. Powsand that Mr. Powsand has noticed. Once they agree that something is wrong, the most effective response to anticipatory grief is often to acknowledge it openly. This can provide relief to both Mr. Powsand and his wife, and should be followed by a careful exploration of her feelings and concerns.

A frank discussion with a physician can be supplemented by life-review activities offered by clergy, psychologists, social workers, or others. The goal of a life review is to develop a sense of closure by reviewing meaningful events that the patient and his or her family have shared. Whether it is led by the physician or by a trained hospice provider, a life review can reduce anxiety and help the patient and family members to focus on making the best use of remaining time together. A life review may also help Dr. Wedlich to identify Mrs. Powsand's concerns about future practical problems, such as financial

---

Table 10-1. Terminology.

- **Grief**—the experience of psychological, behavioral, social, and physical reactions to loss of someone or something that is closely tied to a person's identity.
- **Anticipatory grief**—a grief reaction that occurs in anticipation of an impending loss.
- **Mourning**—the process by which people adapt to loss.
- **Bereavement**—the period of time after a loss during which grief is experienced and mourning occurs.
- **Complicated mourning**—delayed or incomplete adaptation to loss.

Adapted from Rando T. Treatment of Complicated Mourning. Champaign, IL: Research Press; and Freud S. Mourning and melancholia. In: Works, vol 20. London: Hogarth Press; 1917.

Table 10-2.   Summary of Interventions and Assessments.

Anticipatory grief
    Encourage open discussion
    Clarify plans for future
    Do life review

Acute grief
    Offer follow-up appointment
    Acknowledge own sense of loss
    Provide time/permission to grieve
    Assess immediate plan

Early (<1 month)
    Elicit concerns about grief symptoms
    Assess social support
    Assess coping resources
    Identify practical/financial problems

Late (>1 month)
    Assess progress of mourning
    Identify depression
    Consider referral for counseling
    Consider pharmacotherapy

difficulties that might follow Mr. Powsand's death. A life review can also help to ease the dying process, and it may also reduce distress after the patient's death (7).

> *During the next 2 months, Mr. Powsand and his wife meet several times with Dr. Wedlich and a social worker. Mrs. Powsand also meets separately with her minister. Although Mrs. Powsand continues to avoid many social activities, she does resume her bridge game and acknowledges that her friends have become a strong source of support. She continues to have crying spells, but she is able to talk to her husband about his death and to discuss plans for the future.*

Acute Grief

> *Mr. Powsand is admitted to the hospital with an acute myocardial infarction and severe pulmonary edema. He becomes*

increasingly hypoxic, confused, and combative. Dr. Wedlich meets with Mrs. Powsand and the couple's two daughters. Together they determine that Mr. Powsand would not have wished to undergo endotracheal intubation and hemodynamic monitoring. Haloperidol is given as needed for agitation, and Mr. Powsand dies peacefully several hours later.

Dr. Wedlich is called urgently to the bedside. Mrs. Powsand and her daughters are all in the room. Mrs. Powsand is extremely distraught, is sobbing uncontrollably, and is preventing anyone from touching or moving Mr. Powsand. She sits on the edge of his bed, facing the wall, repeating: "He's not dead yet, he's not dead yet." The nurses and daughters want Dr. Wedlich to "do something" immediately.

Despite the best efforts of providers, and careful attention to anticipatory grief, some families will experience dramatic and often disturbing acute grief reactions like the one described here. Acute grief reactions may include denial, intense crying spells, anxiety, "numbness," and somatic symptoms (2,8,9) that may be distressing to family and health care providers. The principal challenge that Dr. Wedlich faces at this stage is to overcome his personal discomfort and feelings of awkwardness to provide support.

Dr. Wedlich can do this most effectively by offering his presence. There are no pressing indications for diagnosis or intervention, and he should avoid the all too common impulse to try to "fix" the problem. Simply by sitting in the room with Mrs. Powsand and by being a witness to her expressions of grief, he is providing an invaluable service. Spending a few moments with the family in silent contemplation and support are by far the most important "interventions."

Dr. Wedlich can provide support in other ways. For instance, he can express his feelings for Mr. Powsand in a way that is both honest and natural by saying that he was honored to have known him, or simply that he will be missed. In addition, he can compassionately and gently confirm that the patient is dead. He can do this as he acknowledges her grief, by saying, "I'm sorry that he is gone."

Dr. Wedlich can also support other family members by acknowledging that Mrs. Powsand's response is disturbing to them and by assuring them that it is not abnormal. It may also be useful to explain that Mrs. Powsand does not mean literally that her husband is still alive.

Instead, her apparent denial may be her way of expressing the sense of loss that they are all feeling.

Additionally, Dr. Wedlich can offer to call a hospital chaplain or the bereaved's own clergyman. He can also give the family the opportunity to grieve by arranging time alone with their loved one's body. Dr. Wedlich can also give Mrs. Powsand and her family "permission" to grieve by suggesting that the next hours and days will be very difficult and that the bereaved may wish to reduce other commitments. This sort of "anticipatory guidance" can provide immediate support, and it can help the bereaved to anticipate and recognize difficulties in the future.

This process may be somewhat easier for Dr. Wedlich because he has established a relationship with the patient and his wife. This ideal may not be achieved in many settings, and some patients will die in the presence of providers they have never met. Nevertheless, all of the interventions described above are equally appropriate and perhaps even more important when a patient dies among strangers.

Before he leaves the bedside, Dr. Wedlich should attend to several practical matters. First, he should be sure that Mrs. Powsand has a way to get home from the hospital, and that she will have a companion for the next several days. Second, he should also arrange a follow-up appointment for her. This appointment should be in 1 or 2 weeks, and should ideally be with Mrs. Powsand's primary physician. However, it may also be with Dr. Wedlich, depending on her preference and the relationship she has established with each. Even if this visit cannot be provided as a billable service, it is important that it occurs.

Dr. Wedlich should offer a condolence contact. This contact should be a telephone call but may be a handwritten note, which can give other providers a chance to extend their condolences as well. This brief contact is important, and it can be a significant source of comfort to the bereaved (10). Physicians may find it helpful to develop a reminder system to ensure that contact is made (11).

Dr. Wedlich should also consider attending the funeral or memorial service. Although he may feel uncomfortable doing so, his presence can provide an opportunity for his own personal healing and can offer comfort to the bereaved. This is a personal decision that should depend on the relationship with the deceased and his or her family. Nevertheless, physicians should strongly consider attending.

Dr. Wedlich spent time with Mrs. Powsand and her family at the bedside. Mrs. Powsand gradually became calmer but refused to allow the nurses to remove Mr. Powsand's body. Dr. Wedlich asked Mrs. Powsand whether she would be willing to help the nurses wash and prepare the body, and she agreed. This seemed to help her to acknowledge his death, and she allowed the body to be removed. She agreed to see Dr. Wedlich in follow-up, then left to spend the night with one of her daughters.

Normal Grief

Dr. Wedlich discusses the follow-up plan with her primary physician and arranges for an appointment in 2 weeks. During that visit, she reports that she has been unable to concentrate on her housework or shopping and is bothered by the state of her house. She has been staying with her younger daughter for the past 2 weeks and feels "at loose ends." She also describes a frequent sensation that her husband is present in the room with her. When Dr. Wedlich asks how she spends her days, she says, "I just sit and look around the room, or I go back to our house and wander around, picking things up and putting them back."

Mrs. Powsand is experiencing grief that is "typical" in the sense that its manifestations are unique to her. Not all people experience all manifestations of grief nor do they experience them in a predictable order. Although Mrs. Powsand is concerned about the time course of her mourning, Dr. Wedlich should emphasize that 2 weeks is not adequate time to assess the progress of bereavement. Instead, he should evaluate the symptoms that Mrs. Powsand is experiencing and determine if they are to be expected and appropriate or are extreme and interfering with her life. He can do this by asking four to five brief, open-ended questions (Table 10-3).

This interview should include a discussion of the symptoms of grief, which are numerous and varied, and may be distressing (Table 10-4). For instance, Mrs. Powsand's perception of her husband's presence may lead her to wonder whether she is suffering from a psychiatric illness. Dr. Wedlich should recognize the grief responses that Mrs. Powsand has experienced and should identify those that are most troubling or that concern her the most. He can respond by acknowledging

Table 10-3. The Brief Bereavement Interview.

Responses to grief
"You've faced a lot over the past several weeks. How has that been for you?"
"How have things been different for you?"
"Is there anything that has been especially troubling to you?"

Social support
"Has anyone been particularly helpful to you in the last month?"

Coping resources
"Are there any activities that have made this less difficult for you?"

Practical difficulties
"How are things around the house? With your finances?"

Table 10-4. Manifestations of Grief.

Psychological Symptoms	Physical Symptoms
Sadness	Anorexia
Anxiety	Change in weight
Helplessness	Trouble initiating/maintaining sleep
Emotional lability	Fatigue
Irritability	Headache
Apathy	Palpitations
Disbelief	Hair loss
Impaired concentration	Grastrointestinal distress
Lowered self-esteem	
Hallucinations of deceased's presence (visual or auditory)	
Feelings of unreality	
Numbness	
Denial	
Searching for the deceased	

Adapted from Rando T. Treatment of Complicated Mourning. Champaign, IL: Research Press; 1993:36-9.

her concerns and by reassuring her that such symptoms are to be expected and are appropriate.

In some instances, however, when cultural differences exist, it will be the bereaved who reassures and educates the physician. For example, among the Navajo, tradition expects that the bereaved express grief only during the 4-day period after death (12), which may be surprising to many physicians. Understanding specific cultural expectations like this would be helpful, but most clinicians do not possess such in-depth knowledge. Therefore, it is important that the physician ask the bereaved or other family members about special customs, beliefs, or cultural norms.

In assessing Mrs. Powsand's grief, Dr. Wedlich should also identify deficits in social support, which are associated with prolonged or difficult grief (13-15). Even if Mrs. Powsand had a strong system of social support at the time of her husband's death, this system may weaken during bereavement if friends and family withdraw because they feel awkward. In addition, Mrs. Powsand may feel uncomfortable going to social events alone, or she may withdraw from these activities altogether.

As Dr. Wedlich gathers this information, he can work with Mrs. Powsand to identify coping resources that she has found to be comforting. She may find that spending time with family or friends is helpful, or she may focus on housework or other activities. She may also find comfort in creating a memorial to her husband in the form of a scrapbook, a charitable donation, or a scholarship in his name. Dr. Wedlich can help Mrs. Powsand to review these coping strategies and can encourage her to make use of those that offer her comfort.

Finally, Dr. Wedlich can also help Mrs. Powsand solve the practical problems that arise now that she is alone. These difficulties may be particularly pronounced in elderly couples, who are often dependent upon one another for financial and domestic tasks of daily life, such as balancing a checkbook. In many situations, referral to a social worker may be needed.

Dr. Wedlich reassures Mrs. Powsand that her feeling that her husband was still present was normal and did not indicate a psychiatric illness. She says that although close friends in her bridge club provided support before Mr. Powsand's death, she was reluctant to return because she thought it would seem inappropriate for her to go out socially so soon after his death. Dr. Powsand acknowledged her concerns but encouraged her to continue to draw on the sources of support that she had found helpful in the past.

Complicated Grief

Four months after Mr. Powsand's death, Mrs. Powsand's daughter calls Dr. Wedlich to say that her mother has been feeling tired and "lethargic." She feels that this has been going on since Mr. Powsand's death. However, she notes that these symptoms became much worse a month ago but have improved somewhat since then. Mrs. Powsand has been spending most of her time in the house and been reluctant to return to activities that she had found pleasurable in the past. Her daughter asks Dr. Wedlich for "something to help Mom's mood."

Mrs. Powsand is experiencing fatigue and anhedonia, and has been withdrawing from her usual activities. These responses may be features of normal grief, or they may be indications of complicated grief. Complicated grief, including depression, can be understood as a failure to return to pre-loss levels of performance or states of emotional well-being (13). Because both depression and complicated grief are indications for additional counseling or psychotherapy, Dr. Wedlich should arrange a follow-up visit.

At this visit, Dr. Wedlich should rule out organic causes for Mrs. Powsand's symptoms, and should determine whether her grief is complicated. Although the distinction between normal and complicated grief is rarely straightforward, several guides can be useful. First, in considering the possibility of complicated grief, Dr. Wedlich should look for evidence of depression. Overall, estimates of depression in the first year of bereavement range from 17% to 27% (16), and suicidal ideation is present in up to 54% of bereaved, even 6 months after the death (17-19).

Physicians may find it difficult to distinguish grief from depression because feelings of guilt, thoughts of death, and psychomotor retardation can be features of both (20). However, symptoms caused by depression typically begin later, after 1-2 months of bereavement (21). In addition, depression is more likely when somatic signs and symptoms persist several months after the loss (21,22). Finally, depression is more likely when symptoms are constant (22). Conversely, symptoms caused by grief often become worse in response to identifiable events or cues, such as holidays or anniversaries. None of these criteria is absolute. But taken together, they should prompt consideration of antidepressant therapy and/or referral to a psychiatrist.

In this case, Mrs. Powsand is unlikely to have depression because her symptoms of lethargy and sadness have been present since her husband's death. Furthermore, they are accompanied by few if any somatic symptoms such as a change in appetite, weight, or sleep. Finally, her feelings of sadness and apathy have waxed and waned over time, with an identifiable exacerbation on her 30th wedding anniversary.

However, Mrs. Powsand still may have complicated grief. Complicated grief may be very difficult to define because the experience of grief is so variable among individuals (23,24). Moreover, the experience of grief tends to relapse and remit over time. For instance, C. S. Lewis wrote of his own experiences with grief that: "One keeps on emerging from a phase, but it always recurs. Am I going in circles, or dare I hope I am on a spiral?" (25).

Despite these challenges, one useful clue to complicated grief can be found in a history of risk factors. For instance, grief may be more pronounced and more distressing in younger people (26-28), women (29-31), and in those with low social support (13-15). Grief may also be more difficult when a death was sudden or traumatic (32). The presence of any of these features should alert the physician to the possibility of complicated grief.

Dr. Wedlich should also look for indications of complicated grief in the course that bereavement takes. For instance, Rando (1) suggests that there are six distinct processes of mourning (Table 10-5). Initially, Mrs. Powsand must recognize the loss of her husband. She should adjust her life accordingly and begin to confront the loss emotionally. Finally, she should seek new relationships and pursuits. It is important to note that the result of these processes is accommodation, not acceptance. Accepting and overcoming a loss is not always a realistic goal, nor is a failure to do so a sign of abnormal grief. For many people, a more realistic aim is a revised life in which the deceased is integrated (1).

These mourning processes have two crucial implications for Mrs. Powsand's case. First, she should not expect to "recover" within a defined period of time, and Dr. Wedlich should reassure her that continued symptoms are not abnormal, if she is making progress in other ways. Second, Dr. Wedlich cannot assess her progress adequately at a single point in time. Instead, he must define the time course of her grief, and how it has changed, in order to determine whether grief is complicated. To do this, Dr. Wedlich may find it helpful to ask focused questions that assess processes of mourning (see Table 10-5).

It seems likely that Mrs. Powsand's mourning has not progressed. In fact, her feelings of sadness and lethargy have persisted with little

Table 10-5.   Complicated Bereavement Interview.

Avoidance
  Recognize the loss
    "Tell me about your husband's death."
    "How was it for you after he died?"

Confrontation
  React to the separation
    "How has his death changed your life? How are you different?"

  Recollect and reexperience the deceased and the relationship
    "Tell me about your husband."

  Relinquish the old attachments to the deceased
    "What do you feel you've lost since he died?"

Accommodation
  Readjust
    "What have you done to help you cope with his death?"
    "How has your life changed since he died?"

  Reinvest in the future
    "What do you think the future holds for you?"
    "What will tell you that you're coping well?"

Adapted from Rando T. Treatment of Complicated Mourning. Champaign, IL: Research Press; 1993:45.

improvement. For people whose grief does not develop toward accommodation, several therapeutic options are available.

One is the use of antidepressant therapy. Although data do not support the use of any agent when depression is not present, many clinicians find tricyclics or serotonin reuptake inhibitors to be beneficial. Given this possible benefit, and the benign side effect profiles of most of these agents, a trial of pharmacological therapy is reasonable.

Another option is referral for counseling. Data, though conflicting at times, suggest that a variety of interventions are effective (33). For instance, individualized counseling by a trained volunteer is available in many settings, and there is some evidence to support its efficacy (34,35). Individualized professional counseling is another option that bereaved people may wish to consider (36). Other options include a peer-led support group, or a support group with a leader, in which members share experiences. Both formats have evidence to support their use (37-40).

In summary, the data about these different approaches to therapy are mixed and often contradictory. Therefore, referrals for specific therapies will depend largely on the goals of the bereaved. Referral will also depend upon the availability of services in the bereaved's community and on the provider's familiarity with the available options, so it is reasonable to describe several options. Dr. Wedlich should advise Mrs. Powsand to consider these options and might suggest that she participate in a session with several groups or therapists before making a decision.

Dr. Wedlich should also continue to follow her at monthly or bimonthly intervals until her course has become clear. For bereaved people who experience uncomplicated grief, a single follow-up visit is usually sufficient. However, for those like Mrs. Powsand who are treated with antidepressants or referred for counseling, additional follow-up visits are required. As noted above, these should usually be with the bereaved's primary physician. However, as in this case, the bereaved's preferences should be considered.

Dr. Wedlich discussed several therapeutic options, and Mrs. Powsand decided to see a psychologist that her minister recommended. She sees Dr. Wedlich again 2 months later and reports that she feels less fatigued. She still misses her husband very much and feels his presence occasionally. However, she is looking forward to the impending birth of her first grandson, who will be named after Mr. Powsand.

Summary

The care of the bereaved is challenging because few data and landmarks distinguish what is normal from what is abnormal. It is challenging, too, because the course of bereavement usually fails to follow a predefined trajectory, and leaves the bereaved and physician unsure of the future. For all of these reasons, as well as the discomfort and uncertainty that can accompany conversations about death and dying, bereavement poses challenges that many physicians may find daunting.

But the care of the bereaved offers opportunities as well. For instance, physicians can gain valuable insight into the natural processes of healing that put end-of-life care, and medical practice, in perspective. To care for dying patients, physicians must understand that the wounds of loss and grief can heal with time. With this knowledge, earned through experience, physicians will be better able to take on the challenges of end-of-life care.

With this knowledge, physicians will also be better able to care for themselves. Although this case focuses on a patient and his widow, it is important to emphasize that grief is by no means limited to the families and friends of patients who have died. Physicians, nurses, and other health care workers often mourn the loss of a patient, and at times the sense of grief can be profound and even temporarily disabling. The assessment strategies and the interventions described here are equally appropriate for health care providers. Therefore, physicians should always consider the possibility that they and their colleagues may also be grieving, and they should be prepared to seek support and to offer it as well.

Attention to bereavement offers a valuable opportunity to participate in healing in its purest form. It is an opportunity to leave technology behind for a moment, and to heal by listening, with words, and with gestures. Physicians have few opportunities to touch lives as profoundly as they can by being present at a patient's death, or by attending a funeral. It is a rare chance to be a doctor, in the original sense of teacher, and to help a patient through a difficult time of tragedy and personal growth. The opportunity to help a patient through the period of bereavement is an opportunity that should not be missed. Bereavement should be an integral part not only of end-of-life care but of all medical practice.

Acknowledgements

Dr. Casarett is supported by a Research Career Development Award in Health Sciences from the Department of Veterans Affairs.

REFERENCES

1. **Rando T.** Treatment of Complicated Mourning. Champaign, IL: Research Press; 1993.
2. **Parkes CM**. Bereavement: Studies of Grief in Adult Life. London: Tavistock; 1972.
3. **Helsing KJ, Szklo M.** Mortality after bereavement. Am J Epidemiol. 1981;114:41-52.
4. **Eliot TD.** Bereavement as a problem for family research and technique. The Family. 1930;11:114-15.

5. **Rush B.** Medical Inquiries and Observations upon the Diseases of the Mind. Philadelphia: Kimber and Richardson; 1812.
6. **Theut SK, Jordan L, Ross LA, Deutsch SI.** Caregivers' anticipatory grief in dementia: a pilot study. Int J Aging Hum Dev. 1991;33:113-8.
7. **McCorkle R, Robinson L, Nuamah I, et al.** The effects of home nursing care for patients during terminal illness on the bereaved's psychological distress. Nurs Res. 1997;47:2-10.
8. **Bowlby J.** Sadness and Depression, vol. 3. London: Hogarth Press and Institute of Psychoanalysis; 1980.
9. **Lindemann E.** Symptomatology and management of acute grief. Am J Psychiatr. 1944;101:213-18.
10. **Tolle SW, Bascom PB, Hickam DH, Benson JAJ.** Communication between physicians and surviving spouses following patient deaths. J Gen Intern Med. 1986;1:309-14.
11. **Abrahm JL, Colley M, Ricacho L.** Efficacy of an educational bereavement program for families of veterans with cancer. J Cancer Educ. 1995;10:207-12.
12. **Miller SI, Schoenfeld L.** Grief in the Navajo: psychodynamics and culture. Int J Soc Psychiatr. 1973;19:187-91.
13. **Prigerson HG, Frank E, Kasl SV.** Complicated grief and bereavement-related depression as distinct disorders: preliminary empirical validation in elderly bereaved spouses. Am J Psych. 1995;152:22-30.
14. **Sanders CM.** Risk factors in bereavement outcome. In: Stroebe MS, ed. Handbook of Bereavement: Theory, Research, and Intervention. New York: Cambridge University Press; 1993:255-67.
15. **Vachon ML, Stylianos SK.** The role of social support in bereavement. J Soc Issues. 1988;44:175-90.
16. **Jacobs S, Kim K.** Psychiatric complications of bereavement. Psych Ann. 1990;20:314-17.
17. **Byrne GJ, Raphael B.** Depressive symptoms and depressive episodes in recently widowed older men. Internat Psychoger. 1999;11:67-74.
18. **Rosengard C, Folkman S.** Suicidal ideation, bereavement, HIV serostatus and psychosocial variables in partners of men with AIDS. AIDS Care. 1997;9:373-84.
19. **Szanto K, Prigerson H, Houck P, et al.** Suicidal ideation in elderly bereaved: the role of complicated grief. Suicide Life Threat Behav. 1997;27:194-207.
20. **American Psychiatric Association.** Diagnostic and Statistical Manual of Mental Disorders (DSM IV), 4th ed. Washington, DC: American Psychiatric Association; 1994.
21. **Jacobs S, Lieberman P.** Bereavement and depression. In: Cameron O, ed. Presentations of Depression. New York: Wiley; 1987.
22. **Shuchter SR, Zisook S.** The therapeutic tasks of grief. In: Zisook S, ed. Biopsychosocial aspects of bereavement. Washington, DC: American Psychiatric Press; 1987.

23. **Levy LH, Martinowski KS, Derby JF.** Differences in patterns of adaptation in conjugal bereavement: their sources and potential significance. Omega. 1994;29:71-87.

24. **Prigerson HG, Shear MK, Newsom JT, et al.** Anxiety among widowed elders: is it distinct from depression and grief? Anxiety. 1996;2:1-12.

25. **Lewis CS.** A Grief Observed. London: Faber and Faber; 1961.

26. **Vachon ML, Rogers L, Lyall WA, et al.** Predictors and correlates of adaptation to conjugal bereavement. Am J Psych. 1982;139:998-1002.

27. **Ball JF.** Widow's grief: the impact of age and mode of death. Omega. 1977;7:307-33.

28. **Reed MD.** Sudden death and bereavement outcomes: the impact of resources on grief symptomatology and detachment. Suicide Life Threat Behav. 1993;23:204-20.

29. **Jacobs S, Kasl S, Ostfeld A, et al.** The measurement of grief: age and sex variation. Br J Med Psychol. 1986;59:305-10.

30. **Sanders CM.** A comparison of adult bereavement in the death of a spouse, child and parent. Omega. 1980;10:303-23.

31. **Zisook S, Shuchter SR, Lyons LE.** Predictions of psychological reactions during early stages of widowhood. Psychiat Clin N Am. 1987;10:355-68.

32. **Weinberg N.** Self-blame, other blame, and the desire for revenge: factors in recovery from bereavement. Death Studies. 1994;18:583-93.

33. **Woof WR, Carter YH.** The grieving adult and the general practitioner: a literature review in two parts (part 2). Br J Gen Pract. 1997;47:509-14.

34. **Parkes CM.** Evaluation of a bereavement service. J Prevent Psych. 1981;1:179-88.

35. **Cameron J, Parkes CM.** Terminal care: evaluation of the effects on surviving of care before and after bereavement. Postgrad Med J. 1983;59:73-8.

36. **Raphael B.** Preventive intervention with the recently bereaved. Arch Gen Psych. 1977;34:1450-4.

37. **Liberman M, Yalom I.** Brief group psychotherapy for the spousally bereaved. Int J Group Psychother. 1992;42:117-32.

38. **Levy LH, Derby JF, Martinowski KF.** The effects of membership in bereavement support groups on adaptation to conjugal bereavement. Am J Community Psychol. 1993;21:361-81.

39. **Vachon ML, Lyall WA, Rogers J, et al.** A controlled study of self-help intervention for widows. Am J Psychiatr. 1980;137:1380-4.

40. **Nolen-Hoeksema S, Larson J.** Coping with Loss. In: Weiner IB, ed. Personality and Clinical Psychology. Mahwah, New Jersey: Lawrence Erlbaum; 1999.

41. **Freud S.** Mourning and melancholia. In: Works, vol 20. London: Hogarth Press; 1917.

SECTION III

Legal, Financial, and Quality Issues

CHAPTER 11

Legal Barriers to End-of-Life Care: Myths, Realities, and Grains of Truth

ALAN MEISEL, JD • LOIS SNYDER, JD •
TIMOTHY E. QUILL, MD

The 15th of April 2000 marked the 25th anniversary of the commencement of the Karen Ann Quinlan legal case and, with it, the start of much of the public discussion concerning medical treatment at the end of life. Substantial legal, ethical, and clinical consensus exists today about care of the dying (1,2), yet myths and misconceptions persist about what is ethically and legally permissible care (3). Sometimes ethics, clinical judgment, and the law conflict with each other. Patients (or families) and physicians can then find themselves considering clinical actions that are ethically and morally appropriate but that raise legal concerns.

The legal context in which care is provided influences both interventions and outcomes. Liability is on the minds of physicians, who tend to overestimate the risk of malpractice lawsuits (4). For instance, a survey of emergency room physicians revealed that most felt legal concerns should not affect resuscitation practices (78%) but nonetheless they did (94%) (5). Communication by physicians about issues in end-of-life care is a primary concern of family members in the care of a loved one (6,7) and is often found to be inadequate (8,9), a factor associated with increased risk of lawsuits (10,11).

Legal Myths, Realities, and Grains of Truth

Legal myths about end-of-life care can lead to actions that comport with neither legal nor ethical norms or with the norms of good medical practice. Table 11-1 summarizes the current legal myths and realities dis-

Table 11-1. Current Legal Myths and Status.

Myths	Realities
Forgoing life-sustaining treatment for patients without decision-making capacity requires evidence that this was the patient's actual wish.	Such treatment may be forgone if the patient's surrogate relates that this was the patient's actual wish or, in most states, if it was the patient's probable wish. Only a few states require "clear and convincing" evidence of patient wishes. In a few states, it is even permissible to terminate life support with the surrogate's permission when the patient's wishes are not known, if termination of treatment is in the patient's "best interests."
Withholding or withdrawing of artificial fluids and nutrition from terminally ill or permanently unconscious patients is illegal.	Like any other medical treatment, fluids and nutrition may be withheld or withdrawn if the patient refuses them or, in the case of an incapacitated patient, if the appropriate surrogate decision-making standard is met.
Risk management personnel must be consulted before life-sustaining medical treatment may be terminated.	There is no legal requirement that a risk manager be consulted before making end-of-life decisions, though some hospital policies may require it.
Advance directives must comply with specific forms, are not transferable between states, and govern all future treatment decisions, and oral advance directives are unenforceable.	Advance directives, often the best indication of an incapacitated patient's wishes, may guide end-of-life decision-making even if all legal formalities are not met. A living will or surrogate should not be consulted if the patient retains decision-making capacity unless expressly authorized by the patient. Oral statements previously made by the patient can also be legally valid advance directives.

If a physician prescribes or administers high doses of medication to relieve pain or other discomfort in a terminally ill patient, resulting in death, the physician will be criminally prosecuted.	If a patient inadvertently dies from the use of high doses of medication intended to treat pain, the physician has not committed murder or assisted suicide.
When a terminally ill patient's suffering is overwhelming in spite of palliative care, and the patient requests a hastened death, there are no legally permissible options to ease suffering.	Although physician-assisted suicide is illegal in most states, terminal sedation is a legal option to treat otherwise intractable symptoms in the imminently dying.
The 1997 Supreme Court decisions outlawed physician-assisted suicide.	Physician-assisted suicide is currently legal in Oregon. Other states are free to legalize or prohibit it.

cussed in this chapter. In a previous work, from 1991, legal myths prevalent then were identified (12), and Table 11-2 summarizes their current status. Some of those myths have now diminished in importance, others persist, and new ones have emerged, creating ongoing barriers to appropriate end-of-life care. One reason for the new myths is that the scope of the debate about the boundaries of end-of-life care has expanded substantially since the Quinlan case (13), including discussion about aggressive management of pain and other symptoms and the possibility of actively hastening death as a last resort.

We outline herein some of the current myths, realities, and grains of truth in several domains of end-of-life care. Physicians should be aware that state laws and hospital protocols affecting end-of-life care vary, and they should seek legal counsel when needed in particular clinical situations.

Withholding and Withdrawing Treatment

Myth 1: Forgoing Life-Sustaining Treatment for Patients Without Decision-Making Capacity Requires Evidence That This Was the Patient's Actual Wish

REALITY

Life-sustaining treatment for patients without decision-making capacity may be forgone if the patient's surrogate relates that this was the patient's actual wish, but it may also be forgone in most states if it was only the patient's probable wish. In a small number of states, it is even permissible to terminate life support with the surrogate's permission when the patient's wishes are not known, if termination of treatment is in the patient's "best interests" (14).

Confusion about this issue may result from the Nancy Cruzan case in which the United States Supreme Court held that doctors were not obligated to terminate treatment at the family's request but could insist on "clear and convincing evidence" that this was the patient's actual wish. However, the Court did not require that other states adopt this standard (15), which in practice is difficult to meet, and most states have not done so. Rather, the prevalent position in law, ethics, and medical practice is to apply the "substituted judgment standard" under which family members are permitted to make end-of-life decisions on the basis of the patient's probable wishes. Most courts presume that family members will best know whether the patient would want to forgo treatment. In a small num-

Table 11-2. Status of Previously Identified Legal Myths.

Myth	Status
There must be a "law" authorizing the termination of life support.	Existing law supports the termination of life supports in all 50 states for competent patients and for those who have lost capacity if there is consensus among those who care about the patient that it would be the patient's will or in his or her best interests.
Termination of life support is murder, assisted suicide, or suicide.	Termination of life supports is considered to be freeing the patient from unwanted bodily invasion. Death is legally considered to be a result of the patient's underlying disease. The law clearly distinguishes such acts from suicide, assisted suicide, or euthanasia.
A patient must be terminally ill for life support to be stopped.	The law allows any patient to refuse any treatment that he or she does not want, in the interest of protecting bodily integrity, even if that treatment would be life sustaining and the patient is not terminally ill.
It is permissible to terminate extraordinary treatments, but not ordinary ones.	The distinction between ordinary and extraordinary treatments is not relevant as a matter of law or ethics. The patient has the right to terminate any treatment, potentially life-sustaining or not.
It is permissible to withhold treatment, but once started, it must be continued.	Although many clinicians think and feel differently about these types of actions, law and medical ethics treat the withholding and the cessation of life-sustaining treatment as the same.
Stopping artificial nutrition and hydration is legally different from stopping other treatments.	In most states, artificial hydration and nutrition are considered medical treatments like any other.
Termination of life support requires going to court.	The courts generally want clinicans to make these decisions without going to court, provided there is a consensus among those who care about the patient about how to proceed.
Living wills are not legal.	Living wills have legal support in all 50 states, through either legislation or case law.

ber of states, under certain circumstances, treatment may be terminated even if the patient's wishes about life-sustaining treatment are unknown and unknowable, if it is in the patient's best interests to do so.

The best evidence of a patient's wishes about life-sustaining treatment is an advance directive. Yet despite the Patient Self-Determination Act and widespread ethical and legal support for advance directives, less than one-fifth of patients complete one (16). Physicians should encourage competent patients to write living wills and/or make surrogate designations through use of a durable power of attorney for health care. When these measures have not been taken by patients, the default approach common in clinical practice is to go to the closest family members to represent the patient in clinical decision-making when the patient cannot speak for him/herself. This default procedure has been codified in law in about two-thirds of the states (14,17). Even in some states without these laws, courts have concluded that close family members may authorize the termination of life support of an incompetent patient (14).

But this is not to say that end-of-life decision-making when the patient cannot speak for him/herself is simple. Sometimes family members' views (and/or the views of close others) about care conflict with each other, or there is a conflict between family members' views and what is known of the patient's wishes. This can be challenging for clinicians in trying to provide the best care and can create fear of litigation. Decision-making for patients who are incapacitated but not permanently unconscious, such as those with Alzheimer's disease, sometimes raises additional challenges (see Chapter 2).

GRAINS OF TRUTH

1. New York law does require evidence of an incapacitated patient's actual wish to forego treatment. Under some circumstances Missouri, Michigan, and Wisconsin do as well (18,19,20).

2. In states that follow this restrictive requirement, there can be variation among hospitals. At one extreme, the ethically sound decisions of caring families may be overridden by health care professionals for their own legal protection. At the other extreme, families may be "coached" to "remember" conversations with the patient about treatment preferences, undermining the integrity of the process and increasing the risk of family problems with bereavement.

3. If there are differences in family opinion about how to proceed, the wishes of a family member advocating a more aggressive medical approach are likely to be given greater weight, even if not based on evidence about patient preferences. This is because of the perceived belief that the legal risks of continuing treatment are less than those of stopping. The default in favor of aggressive treatment is probably stronger if the patient lacks capacity but is not permanently unconscious and has been unclear about his or her wishes.

Myth 2: Withholding or Withdrawing of Artificial Fluids and Nutrition from Terminally Ill or Permanently Unconscious Patients is Illegal

REALITY
Fluids and nutrition are like any other medical treatment; therefore a physician may withhold or withdraw them if the patient refuses this treatment or, in the case of an incapacitated patient, the appropriate standard (as described in Myth 1) is met.

Since 1983, numerous state courts have given their approval to the withholding or withdrawal of artificial nutrition and hydration to terminally ill and permanently unconscious patients, if authorized by the patient, by an advance directive, or by a close family member or other legally authorized person (14). Legally, the death of the patient results from the patient's underlying condition rather than from the conduct of the persons who withhold or withdraw the nutrition and hydration, so there is no legal liability for the patient's death. The Supreme Court's 1990 Cruzan decision (15) gave qualified approval to this practice.

GRAINS OF TRUTH

1. States with high legal standards (patient's actual wishes) about withholding and/or withdrawing feeding tubes or other life-sustaining therapy may effectively preclude these options from being legally available to patients who have not explicitly refused the particular treatment in question in advance of losing decision-making capacity.
2. Even in states that do not generally require evidence of the patient's actual wishes, nursing homes are often reluctant to permit the withholding or withdrawing of artificial feed-

ing without an explicit statement in a written living will, for fear of being the target of regulatory investigation (21).

Myth 3: Risk Management Personnel Must Be Consulted Before Life-Sustaining Medical Treatment May Be Terminated

REALITY

There is no legal requirement that a risk manager be consulted before making end-of-life decisions though some hospital policies may require it.

The objective of risk management is to minimize legal risk to the institution, not necessarily to advise what is ethically or clinically appropriate for a particular patient or even to provide an objective legal analysis of the particular situation. Thus advice from risk managers will not necessarily yield a desirable clinical or ethical, or even legal, result. When end-of-life care treatment dilemmas loom, consultation with an ethics committee or ethics consultant can be helpful. However, in some health care institutions, risk managers may have significant influence on the advice given in an ethics consultation, especially when there is some legal uncertainty, and they tend to err on the side of overestimating the risk to the institution of allowing the termination of life support (22). Thus, it is useful for physicians to be aware of the law in their state as it applies to end-of-life decisions in considering what is clinically and ethically appropriate for their patients in order to be able to evaluate advice given by risk managers and in ethics consultations.

GRAINS OF TRUTH

1. Even though there is no legal requirement to consult risk management, individual hospitals may have adopted such a requirement through internal procedures.
2. Risk management may give greater weight to the hospital's legal protection than to the ethical, medical, and legal interests of the patient where there is legal uncertainty.

Advance Directives

Myth 4: Advance Directives Must Comply with Specific Forms, Are Not Transferable Between States and, Once Signed, Govern All of a Person's Future Treatment Decisions, and Oral Advance Directives are Unenforceable

REALITY

Advance directives are frequently the best source of information about an incapacitated patient's wishes and therefore should provide guidance in end-of-life decision-making even if they do not comply with all legal formalities.

The myth that advance directives are not legally valid has virtually disappeared in the face of the enactment of authorizing legislation in virtually all states. All have health care power of attorney statutes. All but three have living will statutes, and in those three states without living will statutes (Massachusetts, Michigan, and New York) there are court decisions recognizing their validity (19,23,24).

Many advance directive statutes contain living will or health care power of attorney forms. Health care professionals (and even their legal counsel) sometimes believe that to be valid an advance directive must use this form. Although there are some advantages to doing so, a living will or health care power of attorney that does not strictly follow the statutory form is also valid in most states.

Another misconception about advance directives is that they are not "portable"—that is, they are not enforceable except in the state in which they were executed. Many, but not all, advance directive statutes, contain provisions making advance directives that are valid in the state in which they were written enforceable in the state in which the patient now resides. But even in the absence of such a provision, an out-of-state advance directive, like an oral statement or an advance directive that does not use the state form, still provides the best evidence of the patient's wishes about treatment or about who the patient wishes to serve as his or her surrogate.

The purpose of advance directives, acknowledged in most advance directive statutes, is to guide decision-making after a patient has lost decision-making capacity. Thus, as long as a patient retains decision-making capacity, a living will or the patient's health care surrogate should not be consulted about the patient's health care decisions unless the patient expressly authorizes it.

Oral advance directives—that is, oral statements made by the patient about treatment preferences or designating a health care surrogate before losing the capacity to decide—are also legally valid advance directives (14). These statements should be documented in the patient's medical record when known to health care professionals. Periodic conversations with patients, before a final illness as well as during it, can sometimes be more useful in determining the patient's wishes than a living will, as are discussions about who the patient wishes to have as a surrogate.

GRAINS OF TRUTH

1. Using an official form does have some advantages over other written documents or physicians' notes. The state form, if there is one, carries with it the perception that it is valid, and thus it may be more likely to be implemented, especially if the patient's regular physician is not among those caring for the patient.
2. There can be difficulties in proving that oral statements were, in fact, made and what the specific terms were, especially if there is disagreement among family members. Written advance directives may be more likely to be honored especially if the patient's regular physician, who may know the patient's wishes and be able to give credibility to the family's reports of the patient's wishes, is not involved in the patient's care.

Pain Management and Last Resorts

Myth 5: If a Physician Prescribes or Administers High Doses of Medication to Relieve Pain or Other Discomfort in a Terminally Ill Patient and This Results in Death, the Physician Will Be Criminally Prosecuted

REALITY

If a patient inadvertently dies from the use of high doses of medication intended to treat pain (25), the physician has not committed murder or assisted suicide.

In the 1997 United States Supreme Court decisions about the constitutionality of laws making physician-assisted suicide a crime (26,27), a number of the justices wrote about the use of medications for the relief of pain. Some of the opinions supported the use of pain relief medications even in doses that could hasten death, as long as the physician's intent in administering them is to relieve pain and suffering and not to end the patient's life.

The opinions have been hailed by some as creating a constitutional right to excellent pain management and/or to palliative care (28).

Even if the opinions do not go that far, they do clarify some uncertainties that have long plagued end-of-life decision-making. The first concerns the doctrine of double effect. Physicians have long been concerned that the medications needed to provide adequate pain relief to terminally ill patients carried with them the risk that they could indirectly and accidentally end the patient's life by depressing the patient's respiration, thus subjecting the physician to possible criminal prosecution and other legal sanctions. Though generally overstated and overestimated compared with clinical reality (29,29a), this small risk likely contributes to clinician reluctance to use opioids and to the undertreatment of pain in general.

The traditional response has been that the doctrine of "double effect" should alleviate these concerns. Applied in these circumstances, the doctrine holds that where an intervention is used for a legitimate purpose (e.g., pain relief) but has an unintended effect that would be illegitimate if it were intended (e.g., death of the patient), the physician is not morally responsible for the unintended effect (30).

Although this moral doctrine might have eased physicians' consciences, it should not necessarily have eased their concerns about legal responsibility for the patient's death. Before the Supreme Court's decisions, in most states there was no secure legal basis for believing that the doctrine of double effect would contribute to a valid legal defense if a terminally ill patient inadvertently died from analgesic, sedative, or anxiolytic medications, even if these medications were necessary to treat the patient's condition. Although the Supreme Court's decisions do not provide an airtight legal defense when death accidentally occurs from such medications, they give greater assurance that physicians will not be legally responsible under such circumstances. In addition to the protection afforded by the Supreme Court's opinions, almost half of the states have adopted legislation recognizing a right to adequate palliative care (14,31,32) and confer varying kinds and degrees of legal protections on physicians (33).

GRAINS OF TRUTH

1. The application of double effect is ambiguous, particularly if rapidly accelerating doses are needed to treat a terminal crescendo of pain (34), and the line between intending to actively hasten death and intending to relieve pain and suffering can be hazy. A physician who intends to actively

hasten death may be able to escape legal sanctions by claiming an intent merely to treat pain. On the other hand, the physician who intends to relieve pain and suffering could fall victim to legal sanctions if it is difficult to prove this intent. It is impossible to entirely eliminate the risk of potential prosecution for assisted suicide or even homicide, tort liability for wrongful death, disciplinary action by state licensing authorities, or investigation by the Federal Drug Enforcement Administration or similar state authorities.

2. Although physicians acting in accordance with good medical practice have a strong defense, such investigations can take an enormous psychological and/or financial toll on one's personal and professional life.

3. Although "palliative care" legislation may be an important step in the direction of improving access to adequate pain management and providing protection for physicians prescribing in good faith, these statutes suffer from a number of flaws (35), among them that they do not provide complete immunity from liability and that half the states have not adopted them.

4. The safest legal course, based on a comparison of the current legal risks of underprescribing with the risks of prescribing large doses of opioids frequently needed for intractable pain, may still be to underprescribe, although it is the most morally suspect. However, the risk of malpractice suits and disciplinary action for underprescribing pain medications in the face of intractable pain may be on the increase, which might provide some legal counterbalance for the small risk of being accused of overprescribing these medications (36).

Myth 6: When a Terminally Ill Patient's Suffering is Overwhelming in Spite of Excellent Palliative Care and the Patient is Requesting a Hastened Death, There are No Legally Permissible Options To Ease Suffering

REALITY

Although physician-assisted suicide is illegal in most states, terminal sedation may be a legal option to treat otherwise intractable symptoms in the imminently dying.

Although refusing to declare state bans on assisted suicide unconstitutional, the Supreme Court gave indications of approval of "terminal sedation" with the informed consent of the patient (27,37). Terminal sedation integrates two legally accepted clinical practices: 1) sedation of the patient to unconsciousness or a level that ensures escape from intolerable suffering, and 2) withholding life-sustaining therapy including food and fluids (38-40). Even if sedation risks accelerating death, it is consistent with the doctrine of double effect as long as its primary purpose is to ease the patient's pain, discomfort, and anxiety. (In fact, not only is it legally permissible for physicians to provide sedation during the termination of life support to avoid any pain, discomfort, or anxiety but there is even some legal precedent for the view that sedation must be provided under these circumstances [41-43].). The legal and clinical acceptability of withholding of fluids and nutrition was discussed in Myth 2.

GRAINS OF TRUTH

1. Although the Supreme Court approved of terminal sedation, and each of its two components is legally acceptable, the combination of the two components has never been tested in the courts, and thus its overall legality is somewhat uncertain. There is some debate about whether such practice represents "slow euthanasia" (44) or is simply a combination of standard palliative practices. In legal application, the biggest stumbling block is the physician's intention: whether the relief of suffering (legal) or the active hastening of death (illegal).

2. Clinical, ethical, and legal discussions about terminal sedation are relatively undeveloped compared to other end-of-life practices, and practice guidelines have been proposed (38) but not endorsed by professional organizations, so it is likely to be unevenly available.

Myth 7: The 1997 Supreme Court Decisions Outlawed Physician-Assisted Suicide

REALITY

Physician-assisted suicide is currently legal in Oregon. Other states are free to legalize or prohibit it.

In the 1997 United States Supreme Court cases, terminally ill patients and their doctors in Washington state and in New York state argued that the laws of these states that make aiding suicide a crime were unconstitutional, at least when the adult seeking to end his or her life is competent and terminally ill and when the person providing the assistance is a licensed physician. These challenges failed, with the Supreme Court ruling that laws making aiding suicide a crime do not violate the United States Constitution, and thus there is no constitutional right to what is commonly referred to as "physician-assisted" suicide.

However, the Supreme Court did not rule that states cannot legalize physician-assisted suicide. Thus, although the United States Constitution does not require states to legalize physician-assisted suicide, it also does not prohibit them from doing so. The Court left it up to each state to decide for itself how to address the concerns about physician-assisted suicide, and it gave a green light for states to legalize physician-assisted suicide if they wish.

In 1994, Oregon voters approved such a law by referendum. This law, the Oregon Death with Dignity Act (45), permits a physician to prescribe a lethal dose of medication for a competent, terminally ill person who requests it, which the patient must self-administer. Four months after the United States Supreme Court declined to recognize a constitutional right to physician-assisted suicide, the Court also refused to block implementation of this law (46). About 2 weeks later, Oregon voters reaffirmed their support for the legalization of physician-assisted suicide by 60% to 40%.

The Oregon law allows a physician to write a prescription for, but not to administer, a lethal substance. The law clearly distinguishes this practice from euthanasia, in which the physician would administer the lethal medication at the patient's request. Physicians openly practicing euthanasia are more likely to be vigorously and successfully prosecuted (47), as exemplified by the successful prosecution of Jack Kevorkian for administering a lethal injection to a patient after several unsuccessful prosecutions for helping patients end their own lives.

Because physician-assisted suicide has been legalized only in Oregon, physicians in other states who provide a patient with the means to end his or her own life, knowing that the patient intends to do so, could be subject to criminal prosecution and the imposition of professional discipline. In practice, however, it is an open secret that such conduct sometimes occurs without the imposition of any legal sanctions (48-50).

In no state is it legally permissible for a physician to administer a substance to a patient with the intent to end the patient's life, even at the patient's request or with the patient's consent. However, if the physician's intent is the relief of pain and suffering, and the patient dies as an unintended consequence, there should be no criminal liability under the principle of double effect.

GRAINS OF TRUTH
Despite the Supreme Court's ruling that states are free to legalize physician-assisted suicide, only Oregon has done so. Furthermore, several states that previously had no statute making physician-assisted suicide a crime have subsequently criminalized the practice.

Summary

Although there is much legal and ethical consensus about care of the dying, some confusion and gray areas still remain. Some legal barriers are more mythical than real, but many times there is a grain (or more) of truth in the myth, which is probably one reason that physicians may overestimate the legal risks of some practices. In addition, departures from the consensus exist in individual states, so physicians must know the laws of the state in which they practice.

REFERENCES

1. **Meisel A.** The legal consensus about forgoing life-sustaining treatment: its status and its prospects. Kennedy Institute Ethics J. 1992;2:309-45.
2. **American College of Physicians.** Ethics Manual, 4th ed. Ann Intern Med. 1998;128:576-94.
3. **Solomon MZ, O'Donnell L, Jennings B, et al.** Decisions near the end of life: professional views on life-sustaining treatments. Am J Pub Health. 1993;83:14-25.
4. **Localio AR, Lawthers AG, Brennan, TA, et al.** Relation between malpractice claims and adverse events due to negligence. N Engl J Med. 1991;325:245-51.
5. **Marco CA, Bessman ES, Schoenfeld CN, Keler GD.** Ethical issues of cardiopulmonary resuscitation: current practice among emergency physicians. Acad Emerg Med. 1997;4:898-904.
6. **Hanson LC, Danis M, Garrett J.** What is wrong with end-of-life care? Opinions of bereaved family members. J Am Geriatr Soc. 1997;45:1139-44.

7. **Jacobson JA, Francis LP, Battin MP, et al.** Dialogue to action: lessons learned from some family members of deceased patients at an interactive program in seven Utah hospitals. J Clin Ethics. 1997;8:359-71.

8. **Lo B, Quill TE, Tulsky JA.** Discussing palliative care with patients. Ann Intern Med. 1999;130:744-9.

9. **Tulsky JA, Fischer GS, Rose MR, Arnold RM.** Opening the black box: how do physicians communicate about advance directives? Ann Intern Med. 1998;129:441-9.

10. **Duffy FD.** Dialogue: the core clinical skill. Ann Intern Med. 1998;128:139-41.

11. **Levinson W, Roter DL, Mullooly JP, et al.** Physician-patient communication: the relationship with malpractice claims among primary care physicians and surgeons. JAMA. 1997;277:553-9.

12. **Meisel A.** Legal myths about terminating life support. Arch Int Med. 1991;151:1497-1502.

13. In re Quinlan, 355 A.2d 647 (NJ 1976).

14. **Meisel A.** The Right to Die. New York: John Wiley; 1995. Supplement. New York: Aspen Law & Business; 2000.

15. Cruzan v. Director, 497 U.S. 261 (1990).

16. **Goodman M, Tarnoff M, Slotman J.** Effect of advance directives on the management of elderly critically ill patients. Crit Care Med. 1998;26:701-4.

17. **Orentlicher D.** The limits of legislation. University of Maryland Law Review. 1994;53:1255-1305.

18. Cruzan v. Harmon, 760 S.W.2d 408 (Mo. 1988).

19. Martin v. Martin, 538 N.W.2d 399 (Mich. 1995).

20. Edna M.F. v. Eisenberg, 563 N.W.2d 485 (Wis. 1997).

21. **Meisel A.** Barriers to forgoing nutrition and hydration in nursing homes. Am J Law Med. 1995;21:335-82.

22. **Kapp MB.** As others see us: physicians' perceptions of risk managers. J Healthcare Risk Management. 1996;16:4-11.

23. In re Westchester County Medical Ctr. (O'Connor), 531 N.E.2d 607 (N.Y. 1988).

24. In re Spring, 405 N.E.2d 115 (Mass. 1980).

25. **Quill TE, Lo B, Brock DW.** Palliative options of last resort: a comparison of voluntarily stopping eating and drinking, terminal sedation, physician-assisted suicide, and voluntary active euthanasia. JAMA. 1997;278:2099-104.

26. Washington v. Glucksberg, 521 U.S. 702 (1997).

27. Vacco v. Quill, 521 U.S. 793 (1997).

28. **Burt RA.** The Supreme Court speaks: not assisted suicide but a constitutional right to palliative care. N Engl J Med. 1997;337:1234-6.

29. **Hanks G, Cherny N.** Opioid analgesic therapy. In: Doyle D, Hanks G, MacDonald N, eds. Oxford Textbook of Palliative Medicine, 2nd ed. Oxford Univ Pr; 1997.

29a. **Breitbart W, Passik S, Payne D.** Psychological and psychiatric interventions in pain control. In: Doyle D, Hanks G, MacDonald N, eds. Oxford Textbook of Palliative Medicine, 2nd ed. Oxford Univ Pr; 1997.

30. **Garcia, Jorge L A.** Double effect. In: Reich, WT, ed. Encyclopedia of Bioethics, rev ed. New York: Simon and Schuster/Macmillan; 1995;636-41.

31. **Johnson SH.** Disciplinary actions and pain relief: analysis of the pain relief act. J Law Med Ethics. 1996;24:319-27.

32. **Alpers A.** Criminal act or palliative care? Prosecutions involving the care of the dying. J Law Med Ethics. 1998;26:308-31.

33. **Meisel A.** Pharmacists, physician-assisted suicide, and pain control. Univ Maryland J Health Care Law Policy. 1999;2:201-32.

34. **Quill TE, Dresser R, Brock DW.** The rule of double effect: a critique of its role in end-of-life decision-making. N Engl J Med. 1997;337:1768-71.

35. **Field MJ, Cassel CK, eds.** Approaching Death: Improving Care at the End-of-Life. Washington, DC: National Academy Press; 1997.

36. **Shapiro RS.** Health care providers' liability exposure for inappropriate pain management. J Law Med Ethics. 1996;24:360-4.

37. **Orentlicher D.** The Supreme Court and physician assisted suicide: rejecting assisted suicide but embracing euthanasia. N Engl J Med. 1997;337:1236-9.

38. **Quill T, Byock I.** Responding to intractable suffering: the role of terminal sedation and of voluntary refusal of food and fluids. Ann Intern Med. 2000;132:408-14.

39. **Rousseau P.** Terminal sedation in the care of dying patients. Arch Int Med. 1996;156:1785-6.

40. **Mount B.** Morphine drips, terminal sedation, and slow euthanasia: definitions and facts, not anecdotes. J Palliat Care. 1996;12:31-7.

41. State v. McAfee, 385 S.E.2d 651 (Ga. 1989).

42. McKay v. Bergstedt, 801 P.2d 617 (Nev. 1990).

43. Bouvia v. Superior Court (Glenchur), 225 Cal. Rptr. 297 (Ct. App. 1986).

44. Billings AJ, Block SD. Slow euthanasia. J Palliat Care, 1996; 12: 21-30.

45. Or. Rev. Stat. ßß 127.800 et seq. (1996).

46. Lee v. Harcleroad, 118 S. Ct. 328 (1997).

47. **Miller FG, Fins JJ, Snyder L.** Assisted suicide compared with refusal of treatment: a valid distinction? Ann Intern Med. 2000;132:470-5.

48. **Asch DA.** The role of critical care nurses in euthanasia and assisted suicide. 1996;334:1374-1402.

49. **Back AL, Wallace J, Starks HE, Pearlman RA.** Physician-assisted suicide and euthanasia in Washington state: patient requests and physician responses. JAMA. 1996;275:919-25.

50. **Emanuel EJ, Fairclough DL, Daniels ER, Clarridge BR.** Euthanasia and physician-assisted suicide: attitudes and experiences of oncology patients, oncologists, and the public. Lancet. 1996;347:1805-10.

CHAPTER 12

Financing Care for Those Coming to the End of Life

JOANNE LYNN, MD, MA, MS • ANNE WILKINSON, PhD • LYNN ETHEREDGE

Death is nature's way of telling you that you have been very sick." The old adage now has new meaning. Until recently, accidents, infectious diseases, and childbirth caused most deaths. Death struck every decade of life nearly equally. In contrast, of the 2.3 million Americans who died in 1995, almost three-fourths were older than 65 (1). An analysis of a sample of 1994–1998 Medicare claims indicates that, during the last year of life, 66% of elderly decedents had some mention of heart disease in their claims (36% had congestive heart failure), 26% had chronic obstructive pulmonary disease, 31% had cancer, 23% had a stroke, and 14% had dementia (1a). These conditions involve a substantial period of increasing disability and serious illness before causing death (2). More than half of Americans die in hospitals (3,4), and the timing of death is often quite uncertain. For one region's deaths, only two-tenths had a definable "terminal phase," whereas about seven-tenths died rather suddenly during prolonged chronic illness (5).

Medical care in the last year of life costs about 11% of the health care budget and 27% of Medicare funds (6). Although that proportion of Medicare has held constant for two decades (6,7), the costs during the last year vary by illness and by region (8,9). The current expenditures may be justifiable. These patients are truly "sick enough to die." However, patients, families, and even providers often find the care now provided to be inappropriate or unwanted. The SUPPORT project enrolled 9,105 very sick hospitalized patients, identified problems in their care, and tried and failed to correct those problems (10). In SUPPORT, family members reported that half of those who were conscious near death had moderate-to-severe pain most of their last few days. Patients and their physicians did not routinely make plans for end-of-life care or predictable complications, nor did they discuss the overall course and aims of care. Despite long-term chronic illness with a predictably fatal course, physicians usually considered an order to forgo resuscitation only in the patient's last few days.

Health care providers and payers have become accommodated to compartmentalization and fragmentation of services (11). Typically, physicians direct care in the hospital, and nurses or rehabilitation specialists often control post-hospital skilled care. Social workers and small businesses typically arrange non-professional community care services. Regulations bar hospice, the only program specifically designed to serve patients at the end of life, from integrating services, providers, or financing with the larger acute and long-term care programs. Financing arises from disparate sources: Medicare, Medicaid, private insurance, states (e.g., through the Older Americans Act programs and social services block grants), the Department of Veterans Affairs, and out-of-pocket spending by patients and families. Each funder pays each provider and program under a different set of rules and rates, which are often inconsistent or contradictory (12).

Within this disjointed system, everyone has a story to tell. Often they are stories of unrelieved pain, lost advance directives, ineffective communication, and other serious distress. When describing a good period at the end of life, the storyteller feels obliged to observe that his or her family was "lucky," a description that evidences the serious lack of dependability in care services. Dying people and their families are increasingly dissatisfied with the fragmentation, compartmentalization, inefficiency, unreliability and insensitivity of their care systems. Many efforts are underway to improve care for those coming to the end of life: for example, national professional education efforts (e.g., the end-of-life care consensus panel paper series in the *Annals of Internal Medicine,* sponsored by the American College of Physicians-American Society of Internal Medicine, and EPEC, the Project for Education for Physicians on End-of-life Care, the American Medical Association's educational effort for physicians), basic science research (e.g., the National Institute of Health's recent initiatives), quality improvement initiatives (e.g., the Improving End-of-Life Care Quality Improvement Collaborative) (13), public education (e.g., the Last Acts Campaign, sponsored by the Robert Wood Johnson Foundation), pain control initiatives (14), bereavement support, and more. Substantial successes have already been reported (5,13-16).

However, Medicare payment arrangements continue to create serious financial disincentives and disadvantages for providers who wish to deliver good care. Given the successes occurring in professional education and improved treatments, payment and coverage policies are becoming the most serious impediment to effective reform. This article illuminates how some shortcomings of current care originate in Medicare payment and coverage policies, then explores some possible reforms.

CASE 12-1, PART I. THE SMITHS IN ORDINARY CARE

Mary Smith, 78 years old, faced osteoporosis, diabetes, lack of cardiopulmonary reserve, cataracts, and newly diagnosed breast cancer with lymph node involvement. Her 84-year-old husband was disabled and mentally impaired from a stroke. Social Security provided their only income. They owned only a small house and an old car. Their two children lived in distant cities. Mrs. Smith stopped activities outside of her home 10 years ago when her husband had his stroke. With her surgery, chemotherapy, and radiation treatment, life became quite a struggle. Their children visited but felt overwhelmed and unsure of what to do. Mrs. Smith hired some help when she felt desperate. Sometimes they did not have money for food and medicines. Some volunteer organizations helped occasionally with transportation to doctors' appointments and with equipment loans.

Although her doctor thought they were "getting by," Mr. Smith developed a contracture of his hip and a decubitus ulcer of his sacrum. Mrs. Smith felt terrified and alone and did not get much sleep. Neither of them got any exercise or had friendly contacts. Mr. Smith fell, and Mrs. Smith had to call the fire department to lift him back into bed. Within a week, Mr. Smith could no longer get up to a commode. He went to a nursing home. A few weeks later, Mrs. Smith was brought to the emergency room delirious and dyspneic with a myocardial infarction. Thereafter, she barely had the energy to dress herself and go to the toilet.

Mrs. Smith and her husband now both qualified for Medicaid, which paid for an aide at home for her, for 3 hours, 5 days a week. Hospice declined to enroll her because her survival time was too uncertain for the 6-month expected survival requirement. She could no longer drive, so she could visit her husband only every week or two by cab, a trip that left her exhausted. Her weekends were spent alone watching television in her housecoat and eating the cold sandwiches left by Meals on Wheels each Friday.

When her back became painful a few months later, Mrs. Smith took to bed and became quite constipated. The aide insisted on having a nurse visit, but Mrs. Smith would not go to the hospital or her doctor's office, and her physician would not come to her home. During the days of this impasse, Mrs. Smith became delirious and was then taken to the emergency room with dehydration and constipation.

Mrs. Smith was moved to a different nursing home from her husband a week later, and they each died during one of a series of acute hospitalizations for fever, 3 and 6 months thereafter. Proceeds from the sale of the house covered about half of their accumulated personal debts. Their children felt bitter, guilty, and confused. Mrs. Smith never talked with anyone about her life's meaning or about her thoughts on dying. Although a lifelong churchgoer, she never saw a chaplain or minister as she came to the end of her life. During the 2 years covered in their story, she and her husband had a dozen different doctors. None of them ever saw the Smiths at home. At every change in the location of their care, another doctor took over, only to disappear with the next transfer. Neither patient had a Do Not Resuscitate order until the last few days of their last hospitalization.

No one doubts that stories like this are commonplace, but how does this case turn on financing? Some will say that the shortcomings here arise from inattention by specific providers, denial of death, marginalization of the elderly in the current health care system, the Smiths' personal finances, and so on. Although these contribute to the difficulties experienced by persons like the Smiths, better end-of-life care cannot become routine unless the financing for such care also changes. To illuminate the problem, consider the possibility of an alternative story.

CASE 12-1, PART II. THE SMITHS IN OPTIMAL CARE

Mr. and Mrs. Smith's situation triggered referral to a nurse care coordinator who launched comprehensive, family-centered, service planning. This "preventive" planning came to include plans for hospital use, resuscitation, nursing home use, and financial issues. The care coordinator contacted the Smiths' church, which pitched in with friendly visitors and respite help during her treatment. With home care services, Mr. Smith stayed at home to the end of his life. After his death, Mrs. Smith sold her house and car and moved to an assisted living center near her daughter. She died there a year later, probably from heart disease. She became a regular member of the reminiscence group at the assisted living center. She told her son-in-law, just a few weeks before her death, "My bags are packed and I am ready to go on the trip of my life." She, too, was never again hospitalized, and the family had only two physicians during this time, one in each city.

Events do sometimes unfold in this way, but not often. If one could, one would choose this story. The improved course does not eradicate the anguish of coming to the end of life; it just ensures physical comfort and honors the humanity of the patient and family. How does Medicare financing discourage the services that made the second story possible? Table 12-1 presents estimates of service delivery costs, Medicare reimbursements, and the resulting estimated provider net income for the Smith's ordinary course of care as well as for the optimal course. Prescription drugs and Mrs. Smith's treatments for breast cancer are not included because their effects are about the same in both courses of care. Under each of the two scenarios (the "ordinary" course and the "optimal" course), the first column presents estimated "costs of production" (i.e., what staff time, skills, and supplies cost the

Table 12-1. Hypothetical Medicare Reimbursements and Balance for the Smiths' Ordinary Course and for their Optimal Scenario (in Dollars).*

Service	Ordinary Course			Optimal Course		
	Production Cost	Medicare Payment	Provider Net Income[†]	Production Cost	Medicare Payment	Provider Net Income[†]
Home nursing visits	200	210	10	3,000	2,300	(700)
Physician office visits	600	350	(250)	100	120	20
Physician home visits	0	0	0	1000	450	(550)
Physician hospital visits	2,000	2,300	300	0	0	0
Care coordination	0	0	0	3,000	500	(2,500)
Hospitalizations	20,000	21,000	1,000	0	0	0
ER and ambulance	1,500	2,000	500	0	0	0
Total	24,300	25,860	1,560	7,100	3,370	(3,730)

*We have estimated amounts from our experience and from published tables of Medicare reimbursements. Estimates exclude costs that are not generally covered by Medicare, such as nursing facility, home health aide, and assisted living facility costs.
[†]Provider net income is the difference between the payments and the costs of production, which include "salary" costs for the professionals.

provider). This is not what the provider would "charge" but what the services cost to produce, including salaries and overhead. The second column presents an estimate of current Medicare reimbursement for the service. The third column estimates the net income of each provider type as the difference between the cost of production and the reimbursement by Medicare. The estimates given in Table 12-1 represent estimates by experienced clinicians of their typical costs and payments, although actual reimbursements would vary by case specifics, local practices, and fiscal intermediary policies. However, the overall implications are so substantial that they would not change with other assumptions and estimates within a broad range.

Table 12-1 illustrates how improved care could cost the Medicare program much less than current practice (estimated $25,860 vs. $3,730). Even if Medicare payments were expanded to cover currently uncovered costs, they would amount to just $7000 for the improved course of care. Reducing acute illnesses and hospitalization could yield major savings, in part because the Smiths would receive care coordination, home nursing, and physician home visits. However, not a single health care provider ends up with a better financial return with the improved approach. Only the physician's office/clinic even exceeds the costs of care delivery. Nevertheless, physicians' financial return is better overall in the current payment pattern because hospital visits pay better than home visits. Moreover, Medicare does not pay for the care coordinator, a fundamental element in the better outcome for the Smiths. Although studies of community-based case management for the frail elderly have reported few cost savings (17), targeting patients as needy as the Smiths and better integrating the case management with the primary care physician might offer efficiencies (18). Some health plans have targeted case management for their costliest cases and reported dramatic health status improvements and cost savings (19-21).

Did the reimbursement system cause the less helpful care that has become "ordinary"? Probably not, because the fragmentation of care and the emphasis on hospital treatment antedates Medicare. However, Medicare's payment and coverage policies certainly deter reform and reinforce current practices. Cases like the Smiths are commonplace, and so is the perception by most providers that coordinated, comprehensive care would reduce their financial viability. Medicare does not pay enough to support counseling, planning, and continuity, yet Medicare pays well for hospitalizations, emergency transport, and procedures. Medicare fee-for-service providers have their best financial return by responding to crises, not by preventing them. Indeed, no provider can provide excellent care and pay their own bills with patients like the Smiths. Excellent care cannot depend upon cross-subsidization, charity, or altruism. Providers must be able to make a living providing appropriate services.

Medicare Financing

In fiscal year 1996, about 9% of Medicare payments went to capitated managed care, 2% went to administration, and the remaining 89% covered fee-for-service benefits (including hospice) (22). Medicare pays for care of serious and eventually fatal illnesses in four ways:

1. Fee-for-service payments to various providers (including bundled payments for hospitalizations and for skilled nursing facility days)
2. Per diem payments to hospice providers
3. Monthly capitation payments to managed care plans
4. Monthly capitation payments to PACE, the Program of All-Inclusive Care of the Elderly

Fee-for-Service (Basic) Medicare

Basic Medicare covers diagnosis and treatment of illness as determined by medical necessity and as given by a variety of providers. Medicare does not generally cover "unskilled" custodial care or outpatient prescription drugs. Medicare pays hospitals a fixed amount based on each patient's reason for admission. Medicare covers limited skilled nursing facility care after a hospitalization, although rapidly rising expenditures resulted in changes under the Balanced Budget Act of 1997 (23). Skilled nursing care will soon have a global per diem payment that depends primarily upon the intensity of rehabilitation services. Medicare reimburses physicians on a fee-for-service basis. About three-fifths of beneficiaries have supplemental insurance to help them meet deductibles, co-insurance, and certain uncovered services (24). Medicaid pays the Medicare premiums and cost-sharing for the one-sixth of Medicare recipients who are poor enough to qualify.

This reimbursement structure does not pay for an interdisciplinary care team, outpatient prescription medications, on-call services, or continuity across time and delivery settings (e.g., home, hospital, nursing home, home care). Medicare also does not pay for self-administered medications or for a case coordinator. In summary, fee-for-service Medicare pays for medical treatments and not for long-term continuity or palliative services, just the reverse of what many dying patients need and prefer.

Medicare Hospice Benefit

Hospice programs provide palliative treatments, medications, personal care, spiritual support, and grief and bereavement counseling for both the patient and the family. The Medicare hospice benefit pays for services to "terminally ill" persons with a life expectancy of 6 months or less. Hospice covers only the services needed for the terminal illness. Hospice serves patients at home whenever possible, and the family is expected to help. Participants must declare themselves willing to forgo "curative" medical treatment for their terminal illness. An eligible patient may usually elect hospice while residing in a nursing home, group home, or assisted living facility (except when Medicare is paying for skilled nursing facility care for the fatal illness).

The patient's personal physician can continue to care for a hospice patient, directly billing Medicare Part B. The hospice receives a daily capitation to cover all costs except physician bills (more than 90% are at the basic home care rate, about $94 per day in 1997) (25). The hospice benefit consists of "benefit periods": two 90-day periods followed by an unlimited number of 60-day periods. The hospice must recertify the patient as eligible at the start of each benefit period. There are three other rates: continuous home nursing, inpatient respite, and inpatient symptom control. Eighty percent of hospice enrollees are Medicare beneficiaries (25).

Hospice programs have demonstrated effective care for people in the last phase of life. However, actual hospice program practices and populations served vary considerably across the country. Hospice serves only about 20% of the dying, for about a month on average (26). In 1995 and 1996, cancer accounted for 70% of admitting diagnoses (27). The requirement of 6 months life expectancy and hospices' general approach to care are most compatible with cancer's trajectory, in which the patient functions well at first, then enters a relatively brief and predictable phase of progressive deterioration (28). In contrast, end of life more often follows the Smiths' course: a slow decline in function, punctuated by periodic life-threatening crises, with widely variable, unpredictable survival time (5). The hospice requirement that at least 80% of care days be in the home also bars hospice for patients who do not have a suitable home and a volunteer family member or privately paid caregiver. Finally, patients with organ system failures are less willing to forgo life-prolonging care in a medical crisis because, unlike cancer patients, they often have significant potential for recovery and prolonged survival at close to their previous level of functioning (29,30).

Congress set the Medicare hospice rate when palliative care mainly required opioid medications, personal care, and nursing services. Since then, services for home use have become expensive, such as costly methods of pain relief (e.g., intravenous or intrathecal medication), palliative chemotherapy, infusion of intravenous inotropes, and home positive pressure breathing. Hospices will have financial losses if they admit persons who are likely to want those treatments. Thus, hospice access is limited by various considerations: patients need a predictable 6-month or less life expectancy, patients must explicitly forgo life-prolonging (i.e., "curative") treatments, the traditional focus of hospice is on cancer patients, hospices seek to limit risk in taking expensive patients, and hospice usually requires having a home and a volunteer family caregiver. Although no reasonably current and rigorous research evaluates hospice performance and value, practitioners generally agree that hospice probably serves its traditional patient population well. However, hospice under the Medicare program cannot usually serve patients like the Smiths reliability.

Capitated Managed Care in Medicare

Serving about 15% of the Medicare population (22.5% in urban areas and 0.6% in rural areas) (23,31), capitated plans have both the flexibility and the direct financial incentive to provide cost-effective care and keep patients out of the hospital (32-36).

Managed care plans in the private sector have initiated disease-specific management programs to control utilization and prevent exacerbations for certain high-cost, chronically-ill patients. Descriptions of these programs are mostly unpublished and/or proprietary. However,

Humana Health Care reported a program of intensive case management for congestive heart failure patients who had high emergency room and hospital use and costs ($16.9 million for 1,900 CHF patients nationwide in 1995) (37). Their comprehensive program included telephone case management, an ongoing relationship between the specialist nurse and the patient, patient education, medications, and lifestyle adjustments. Hospital admissions declined 60%; hospital bed days, 58%; hospital costs for congestive heart failure, 78%; and total hospital costs, 68%. Humana also reported that patient sodium intake decreased 20%, functional levels increased 15%, and mortality dropped from an expected 25% to 10% in their first year (1997-1998).

Kaiser-Permanente Bellflower, in California, aimed to tailor care for patients with a prognosis of less than 12 months, homebound status, a deteriorating medical condition at risk of needing symptom control, and a hospital or emergency room visit in the previous year. Most program patients did not want or were not eligible for the Medicare hospice benefit. A "palliative care team" of physicians, nurses, and social workers provided supportive care in the home, supplemented as needed by home health aides, chaplains, volunteers, rehabilitation services, and bereavement support. Telephone support and after-hours home visits were always available. The program usually provided durable medical equipment, prescription medications, and oxygen. The first 19 patients who died in the special program were compared with a control group ($n = 16$) who died in "usual care." In the same time before death, the control group had substantially more acute admissions (15 vs. 6), hospital days (85 vs. 12), intensive care unit days (44 vs. 5), emergency room visits (22 vs. 9), nursing home days (47 vs. 13), and CT/MRI scans (11 vs. 2) than the palliative care patients. The total cost of care for the control group was estimated to be $106,138 versus $36,964 for the palliative care group, with estimated per diem costs of $221 for control group patients versus $72 for palliative care patients (37a).

Unfortunately, managed care plans hesitate to develop such programs. Although cost-effective care to existing members would be a financial advantage, a reputation for excellence in caring for people with complex illness risks attracting people who need expensive care. Medicare pays plans the same amount whether the enrollee is healthy or sick. Thus, plans aim to enroll the healthy and avoid the sick (38-40). Medicare has overpaid capitated plans by an estimated 5% to 20% because of their disproportionately healthy members (41).

The Balanced Budget Act of 1997 will reform the flat payment system (23). To reduce the financial incentives for enrolling healthy persons and to pay more fairly for the care of sick and disabled people, Medicare was to link capitation payments to the health status of beneficiaries by the year 2000 (42). Adjusting payments to reflect the financial risks associated with various conditions should make plans more willing to enroll chronically ill persons and to reimburse physicians more fairly for caring for such persons. Properly calibrated and executed, risk adjustment would allow capitated plans to profit while serving expensive, very sick patients.

However, risk adjustment presents a number of challenges. For example, risk-adjusted payments initially will be set by the previous year's hospitalization diagnoses. Having enhanced payment depends upon hospitalization, contradicting the goals of reducing or preventing exacerbations. Risk adjustment also may not compensate plans adequately for establishing and promoting good care for the chronically ill and dying because they are most often at the high end of costs within each diagnosis. Therefore, capitated providers may not have sufficient confidence to invest in innovative programs or to adopt strategies that attract very sick patients. New risk adjustment payment methods (e.g., mixed capitation, fee-for-service) are being proposed (43).

PACE Model of Improved Care

PACE (Program for All-inclusive Care for the Elderly) is a Medicare program for frail elderly patients who are eligible for nursing home placement. PACE programs offer complete coverage of all Medicare-reimbursed services (including hospital, physician, home health, and skilled nursing home care) and all Medicaid covered services, such as custodial nursing home care, homemaker services, and adult day health care. The Medicare and Medicaid programs each provide a capitated monthly reimbursement. A few patients ineligible for Medicaid pay privately for the Medicaid component (about 8% of enrollees). The Medicare monthly capitation ranged from $689 to $1,562 across PACE sites in 1994. The Medicaid reimbursement rates ranged from $1,486 to $4,465 across sites, with an average of $2,361 (a range of 74% to 95% of each state's nursing home reimbursement rate). The Medicare capitation payment is 2.39 times the local capitation rates for Medicare risk contract group health plans. PACE is now a regular part of Medicare, even though it covers less than 10,000 people.

The most difficult challenge for the PACE program has been enrollment. Whether PACE programs can serve their present enrollees near death or come to serve other populations at the end of life has yet to be tested. Indeed, very little research yet illuminates the effectiveness or costs of PACE in its current form. However, the combined funding and the comprehensive service array are appealing features for end-of-life care.

Summary

Medicare, which provides health care insurance for three-quarters of Americans, has coverage and payment policies in each of its programs that militate against reliable, excellent care.

What Care Should Financial Arrangements Encourage?

Patients facing serious, eventually fatal, chronic illness need a trustworthy, predictable, and effective care system that enables the end of life to be lived in a way that is rewarding and meaningful. Specifically, that care system needs to be reliable enough to make several promises to a patient facing serious chronic illness at the end of life (44):

1. Evidence-based medical and nursing treatment
2. Symptom relief, including assurance that symptoms will never be overwhelming
3. Continuity and comprehensiveness so that no gaps or transfers disrupt care
4. Planning for complications to ensure appropriate care and avoid fear
5. Care customized to match patient and family values, hopes, and concerns
6. Care plans congruent with patient and family resources
7. Assistance to enable the patient to live every day fully

To generate a care system that can promise performance, Medicare financing could encourage at least the following specific characteristics:

1. Continuity of care across care settings and over time
2. Use of evidence-based standards and guidelines
3. Interdisciplinary teams, with responsibility for patient and family care often principally relying upon experienced nurses

4. Mobilization of services to the patient's residence, whether at home, congregate living facility, or nursing facility
5. Education of patient and family in self-management
6. Advance planning of the response to expected urgent situations
7. Quality improvement activities focused upon a defined population and specific problems

What Financial Arrangements Could Encourage Better Care?

Medicare effectively insulates the elderly and most disabled persons from financial ruin from medical treatments and ensures quick access to physicians and hospitals. Reforms should avoid disabling or distorting the valuable features of Medicare. Starting from each of the current programs of payment in Medicare, incremental but substantial reforms are possible.

First, any administratively feasible reform must target a clinically identifiable group who are "coming to the end of life" or "dying." The Patient's Bill of Rights uses a category of "serious and complex" illnesses or "ongoing medical conditions" to trigger various patient protections against abruptly losing a trusted provider (45). However it is named, the category should include those with an illness or condition that will worsen and be fatal, a disability too severe to provide for daily needs, and those with a need for ongoing health care. Rather than being predicated directly upon a statistical claim about prognosis, such a category could turn on indicators of disease severity and disability (46). The population thus identified would have a predictable relationship of survival and time, but any one patient's prognosis could be quite uncertain. Triggering coverage and payment by indices of severity of illness is itself a suitable subject for innovation and demonstration/evaluation projects.

Fee-for-service Medicare could give substantial financial advantage to continuity and comprehensiveness. Once a patient qualifies, care providers with demonstrated excellence in the essential program elements listed above could be paid better than those who continue the current patchwork of disconnected services (16,47). Repeated hospitalizations for the same condition without advance care planning could reduce reimbursement rates. Medicare could require patients with serious chronic disease to designate a provider team for their primary care each year. Provider teams with good performance could also have preferential payments or streamlined administrative procedures (48).

Medicare hospice could expand its scope to serve patients now excluded. For example, the 6-month prognostic criterion could be modified to cover some or all "serious and complex" illness, perhaps with some longer stays being accompanied by lower per diem rates. Some "carve-outs" for high-cost palliative care (medications for AIDS, chemotherapy for pain, neuroablative procedures, etc.) could have enhanced rates. Caring for congestive heart failure patients for a few years, for example, entails different financial risks and strategies than does caring for cancer patients for a few weeks. Appropriate capitation payments to a team dedicated to care of eventually fatal chronic illnesses might offer incentives for reform at controllable cost. Medicare generally precludes hospice providers from consulting in other settings, although their skills are often unique. Medicare reform could relieve that limitation on access.

Capitated managed care in Medicare could protect those with "serious and complex" illness from pre-emptive loss of a long-term provider due to that provider being removed from an authorized provider list. The same patients could have assured access to providers with suitable skills and performance. The risk adjustment for serious and complex illness could start very shortly after identification (rather than with the next fiscal year) and could continue through to the end of life (rather than for a year, unless another hospitalization occurs).

PACE programs might well tailor their services for serious and complex illness such as congestive heart failure or obstructive lung disease. The financing method is well suited to chronically ill populations, and the flexibility and accountability for care are quite attractive. PACE could also establish standards for continuity, advance planning, symptom control, and bereavement support.

Of course, each of these moderate reforms would merit evaluation in demonstration settings or in the early years of implementation. Most reforms yield effects that are different from those anticipated. Thoughtful and effective reform requires ongoing monitoring, insight, and adjustment.

More substantial reforms might be warranted. The Department of Veterans Affairs has recently been quite successful in instituting improvements in end-of-life care across their large system. They have increased the rate of basic advance care planning from about half of those with certain serious diagnoses to more than 90% (48a). They have instituted a system-wide emphasis on pain management. Their structure and budgeting process provides an opportunity to consider alternative investments based on the value for veterans, without short-term effects upon the income for any practitioner or program. Similarly, a budget for other defined populations for a period of time, given to a comprehensive provider program, might yield more reliability, less investment in predictably low-yield (but high-cost) treatments, and more continuity. Indeed, other novel approaches will arise to be tested, if creative minds focus upon the challenge of how to rearrange services and payments to serve the large numbers of persons living with serious and complex, eventually fatal illnesses.

How Is Reform Accomplished?

Public policy change would benefit from a strong and urgent effort to enhance our knowledge about end-of-life care and the systems that could support good care. We need a renewed commitment to innovation, evaluation, and learning about the actual effects of alternative arrangements. Current debates about the future of Medicare focus on paying less for the current system of care, rather than on changing what that system pays for. For the end of life, the care we have now is not what we want to keep purchasing. Reforms that address only the financial solvency of the current Medicare program or enhanced numbers of insured persons will not generally improve end-of-life care. On the other hand, reforming coverage and payment policies so that they encourage providers to serve those with serious and eventually fatal illness will be a particularly powerful and enduring way to improve care at the end of life. Of course, payment and coverage reforms will not be sufficient to ensure good care without simultaneous changes in the skills of providers and the attitudes of society. Nevertheless, Medicare reforms are essential because no one can expect reliably good care to be available if providers cannot make a living by providing the desired services.

Reform will require evidence that a better system can work for patients and families, estimates of each reform's effects on Medicare's costs, and the political will to make improvements despite inertia and resistance. Reformers might build upon the observation that the major pathways to death with serious chronic disease are few, and thus the variety of payment and service arrangements needed is likely to be limited. Reformers also could start with heart and lung diseases, which are currently treated sufficiently aggressively that real savings from more comprehensive and coordinated care are possible (20,49).

Reform requires evidence that better systems of care are within reach. Some of the needed examples of good care arise from quality improvement efforts at the local level, but success also requires widespread implementation in Medicare-sponsored demonstrations. For some desirable outcomes in Medicare, an array of forces seems to be needed to create changed patterns of care. Certainly, other initiatives are addressing some of the impediments to improvement of end-of-life care, such as shortcomings in provider skills and attitudes, and public demand for reliable and competent care is growing. The burgeoning interest in and the early successes of improvement projects that were motivated almost entirely by a devotion to patient service make it plausible that permissive changes in Medicare policy may well enable substantial reform.

However, reform may require that society identify someone to be held accountable for good end-of-life care. At present, everyone involved can feel that they are merely "cogs in the wheel," with no particular obligation to initiate or monitor change. Perhaps Congress could lay responsibility upon a national commission, perhaps at the Institute of Medicine or the Department of Health and Human Services. Perhaps Congress could require annual reports on the state of end-of-life care by the Surgeon General or the Secretary of Health and Human Services. Various strategies could ensure that some enduring groups acknowledge responsibility for accomplishing the aim that Americans be able to count on having good care for the end of life. Only in this way will the necessary data and ideas be presented in a timely and forceful way.

The Smiths' case shows that better care is possible, and it is even possible that good care could cost less. However, financing good care in a fair, sustainable way will require an array of reforms. Financing, to be sure, is only one component. Much work remains to be done to define the population at the end of life and to identify and provide the services most needed. However, unless we simultaneously change Medicare's financing of those services, that work will largely yield no enduring improvements in patient care.

REFERENCES

1. **Field MJ, Cassel CK, eds.** Approaching Death. Washington, DC: Institute of Medicine; 1997.

1a. **Cassel CK, Mologne MK.** VA leadership in pain management and palliative care. Veterans Health System Journal. December 2000.

2. **McMillan A, Mentnech RM, Lubitz JD, et al.** Trends and patterns in place of death for Medicare enrollees. Health Care Financ Rev. 1990;2:1-7.

3. **National Center for Health Statistics.** National Mortality Followback Survey. Vital and Health Statistics, series 20, no. 19. Hyattsville, MD: National Center for Health Statistics; 1994.

4. **Temkin-Greener H, Mieiners MR, Petty EA, Szydowski JS.** The use and cost of health services prior to death: a comparison of the Medicare-only and the Medicare-Medicaid elderly populations. Milbank Q. 1992;70:697-701.

5. **Hammes BJ, Rooney BL.** Death and end of life planning in one midwestern community. Arch Intern Med. 1998;158:383-90.

6. **Lubitz JD, Riley GF.** Trends in Medicare payments in the last year of life. N Engl J Med. 1993;328:1092-6.

7. **Lubitz J, Prihoda R.** The use and cost of Medicare services in the last 2 years of life. Health Care Finance Review. 1984;5:117-31.

8. The Dartmouth Atlas of Health Care. Chicago: American Hospital Publishing; 1996.

9. **Pritchard RS, Fisher ED, Teno JM, et al.** Influence of patient preferences and local health system characteristics on the place of death. J Am Geriatr Soc. 1998;46:1242-50.

10. **The SUPPORT Principal Investigators.** A controlled trial to improve care for seriously ill hospitalized patients. The Study to Understand Prognoses and Preferences for Outcomes and Risks of Treatments (SUPPORT). JAMA. 1995;274:1591-8.

11. **Newcomer R, Harrington C, Kane R.** Managed care in acute and primary care settings. Ann Rev Gerontol Geriatr. 1996;16:1-36.

12. **Weiner J, Skaggs J.** Current approaches to integrating acute and long-term care financing and services. Report 9516. Washington, DC: American Association of Retired Persons; 1996.

13. **Lynn J, Berwick D, Kabcenell A, et al.** Reforming care for those near the end of life: the merits of quality improvement. Submitted to Ann Intern Med.

14. **Du Pen SL, Du Pen AR, Polissar N, et al.** Implementing guidelines for cancer pain management: results of a randomized controlled clinical trial. J Clin Oncol. 1999;17:361-70.

15. **Tolle SW, Rosenfeld AG, Tilden VP, Park Y.** Oregon's low in-hospital death rates: what determines where people die and satisfaction with decision on place of death? Ann Intern Med. 1999;130:681-5.

16. **Lynn J, Schuster JL, Kabcenell A, The Center to Improve Care of the Dying, and The Institute for Healthcare Improvement.** Improving Care for the End of Life: A Sourcebook for Clinicians and Managers. New York: Oxford University Press, 2000.

17. **Wilkinson AM.** Past research on long-term care case management demonstrations. Annu Rev Gerontol Geriatr. 1996;16:78-111.
18. **Fox PD, Etheredge L, Jones SB.** Addressing the needs of chronically ill persons under Medicare. Health Affairs. 1997;17:144-51.
19. **Fonarow GC, Stevenson LW, Walden JA, et al.** Impact of a comprehensive heart failure management program on hospital readmission and functional status of patients with advanced heart failure. J Am Coll Cardiol. 1997;30:725-32.
20. **Rich MW, Beckham V, Wittenberg C, et al.** A multidisciplinary intervention to prevent the readmission of elderly patients with congestive heart failure. N Engl J Med. 1995; 333:1190-5.
21. **MedPAC Commission.** Model programs improving the quality of care. Report to the Congress: Contacts for a Changing Medicare Program. June 1998; p.163.
22. **Welch WP.** What does Medicare pay for? Disentangling the flow of funds to health care providers. Health Affairs. 1998;17:184-97.
23. Public Law 105-33.
24. **Franklin J, Eppig JD, Chulis GS.** Trends in Medicare supplementary insurance: 1992-96. Health Care Finance Review. 1997;19:201-6.
25. **National Hospice Organization.** Hospice Fact Sheet. Arlington, VA: National Hospice Organization; Summer 1998.
26. **Christakis NA, Escarce JJ.** Survival of Medicare patients after enrollment in hospice programs. N Engl J Med. 1996;335:172-8.
27. Hospice Management Advisor. October 1998, p. 118.
28. **Lynn J.** An 88-year-old woman facing the end of life. JAMA. 1997;277:1633-40.
29. **Levenson JW, McCarthy EP, Lynn J, et al.** The last six months of life for patients with congestive heart failure. J Am Geriatr Soc. 2000;48(5 Suppl):S101-9.
30. **Lynn J, Ely EW, Zhong Z, et al.** Living and dying with chronic obstructive pulmonary disease. J Am Geriatr Soc. 2000;48(5 Suppl):S91-100.
31. **Medicare Payment Advisory Commission.** Health Care Spending and the Medicare Program: A Data Book. Washington, DC: Medicare Payment Advisory Commission; 1998.
32. **Morrison DE, Meier DE.** Managed care at the end of life. Trends Health Care Law Ethics. 1995;10:91-6.
33. **Wagner EH.** Population-based management of diabetes care. Patient Educ Counsel. 1995;26:225-30.
34. **Miles SH, Weber EP, Koepp R.** End-of-life treatment in managed care: the potential and the peril. West J Med. 1995; 163:302-5.
35. **Kane RL.** Managed care and older persons: threat or opportunity? In: Managed Care: Making It Work for Older People. Washington, DC: Gerontological Society of America; 1998.
36. **Wilkinson AM, Lynn J, Cohn F, Jones SB.** End-of-life in managed care: achieving excellence through MediCaring. In: Managed Care: Making It Work for Older People. Washington, DC: Gerontological Society of America; 1998.
37. Public Sector Contracting Report. February 1998, pp.24-6.

37a. **Brumley R.** Palliative care: a model of care for seriously ill patients. Presented at Improving Care at the End of Life National Congress. Sponsored by the Institute for Healthcare Improvement and the Center to Improve Care of the Dying. St. Louis, MO; July 1998.

38. **Medicare Payment Advisory Commission.** Report to the Congress: Medicare Payment Policy. Vol. 1. Recommendations. Washington, DC: Medicare Payment Advisory Commission; March 1998.

39. **Riley G, Tudor C, Chiang Y-P, Ingber M.** Health status of Medicare enrollees in HMOs and fee-for-services in 1994. Health Care Finance Review. 1996;17:65-76.

40. **Morgan RO, Virnig BA, DeVito CA, Persily NA.** The Medicare-HMO revolving door: the healthy go in and the sick go out. N Engl J Med. 1997;337:169-75.

41. **Greenwald LM, Esposito A, Ingber MJ, Levy JM.** Risk adjustment for the Medicare program: lessons learned from research and demonstrations. Inquiry. 1998;35:193-209.

42. **Iezzoni LI, Ayanian JZ, Bates DW, Burstin HR.** Sounding board: paying more fairly for Medicare capitated care. N Engl J Med. 1998;339:1933-8.

43. **Newhouse JP, Buntin MB, Chapman JD.** Risk adjustment and Medicare: taking a closer look. Health Affairs. 1997;16:26-43.

44. Developed in the Breakthrough Series Collaborative to Improve Care for Advanced Heart and Lung Failure, sponsored by the Institute for Healthcare Improvement, the Department of Veterans' Affairs, and the Center to Improve Care of the Dying, GWU, January 1999. Available from Americans for Better Care of the Dying via the Internet (http://www.abcd-caring.org). Accessed February 2000.

45. White House memorandum to federal agencies regarding the health care consumer bill of rights and responsibilities. 20 November 1997. Available from White House Press Secretary via the Internet (http://www.pub.whitehouse.gov).

46. **Fox E, Landrum-McNiff K, Zhong Z, et al.** Evaluation of prognostic criteria for determining hospice eligibility in patients with advanced lung, heart, or liver disease. JAMA 1999;282:1638-45.

47. From a Generation Behind to a Generation Ahead: Transforming Traditional Medicare. National Academy of Social Insurance; January 1998.

48. The President's Plan to Modernize and Strengthen Medicare for the 21st Century. The White House (National Economic Council and Domestic Policy Council); 2 July 1999. Available at http://www.whitehouse.gov/WH/New/html/Medicare/toc.html.

48a. **Hogan C, Lynn J, Gabel J, et al.** Medicare beneficiaries' costs and use of care in the last year of life. Final report to the Medicare Payment Advisory Commission. 2000. Washington, DC, MedPAC.

49. **Lynn J, Schall M, Milne C, et al.** Quality improvements in end of life care: insights from two collaboratives. Joint Commission Journal on Quality Improvement. 2000;26:254-67.

CHAPTER 13

Reforming Care for Those Near the End of Life: The Promise of Quality Improvement

JOANNE LYNN, MD, MA, MS • KEVIN NOLAN, MA •
ANDREA KABCENELL, RN • DAVID WEISSMAN, MD •
KATHLEEN CASEY MILNE, RN, CCM, COC •
DONALD M. BERWICK, MD, MPP

CASE 13-1. DR. THOMAS'S STORY

Recognizing a Problem

Dr. Evan Thomas, a hospitalist at General Hospital, was called to the emergency room to admit an 84-year-old woman from a nearby nursing facility. He knew the routine: work-up for fever, then IV antibiotics and fluid balance, and finally either send her back to the nursing facility in a few days or watch over her dying. He was surprised to discover, however, that the patient was Mrs. Harroldson, his high school English teacher some 30 years ago, now shrunken with age and Alzheimer's. He did proceed, perhaps with more tenderness. Mrs. Harroldson had no family, and no one but him seemed to know her from the past. She endured many complications, developed decubiti from fighting restraints, and was barely "hanging on." Dr. Thomas called the nursing home to find a nurse who knew her, but none was available. Mrs. Harroldson had a court-appointed guardian, but that person was a lawyer who did not respond to a voice-mail message. Mrs. Harroldson had a feeding tube inserted and a fruitless resuscitation attempt before she died.

Thereafter, Dr. Thomas was increasingly troubled by his nursing home admissions. Most had no family, and none had made plans about procedures such as resuscitation. Few of the nursing home personnel had any indication about what was meaningful for the patient. He felt himself to be part of an assembly line for fixing the physiology, but realized that these patients could not all have wanted what they got. What was he to do? These patients were one-third of his caseload, but he was no longer sure that his part in their story was of value.

What can Dr. Thomas do? His medical treatment meets the standards of usual practice, but it no longer seems adequate. Dr. Thomas has, nonetheless, taken the first two crucial steps toward improvement. First, he is developing the will to seek improvement because he has concluded that his care falls short in managing symptoms and in advance care planning. Second, he sees that his care pattern affects many patients. These two insights are critical but difficult to achieve. Inattention and accepting the status quo block most opportunities for improvement, and rarely does ferreting out a single error or miscreant yield important improvements. Instead, substantial gains are found in correcting a behavior pattern that affects dozens of patients.

Starting a Process

Dr. Thomas sought some better options. He read professional literature and news articles about programs to serve severely demented people. He talked with the directors of nursing and social workers at two of the best nursing homes in the area. He also talked with experienced geriatricians and followed their leads to other experts. Along the way, he accumulated a list of possible corrective actions: changes that people involved felt might improve things. Most of these turned out to require some agreement about practices and plans among the nursing homes, the emergency medical system, and the hospital-based providers. He decided that his tribute to Mrs. Harroldson's memory would be to bring together a dozen concerned people to see what might be done. At the last minute, he invited the hospital's CEO and the emergency medical technician program director.

Dr. Thomas is doing remarkably well. He has learned about the problem and has assembled a team that cares about it. He has a list of changes to try. He has even started a process to implement change responsibly and effectively. His common-sense approach is quite unusual and exceedingly valuable to his organization. Few people note shortcomings in the system in which they work, see the impact of those shortcomings, think about alternatives, and initiate action. If the CEO is a good leader, she will see that this endeavor is important to support, even though any useful change is likely to cause some uncomfortable disruptions.

Getting Started

The group gathered for supper at his house, mostly meeting one another for the first time. They told stories of shared patients and commented on what they felt worked well and where there were gaps and frustrations. By the end of the evening, they had named their group (The Grey Ladies Coalition), had noted the need to involve some other key players, and had settled on two things to do first: 1) get all health professionals in the area to agree on one way to communicate existing decisions to forgo resuscitation, and 2) assess advance care planning at a quarterly review at one of the nursing homes. The group hoped eventually to involve a wide array of physicians and organizations. They decided, however, to start with those who were eager to be involved. Early successes could fuel enthusiasm.

One nursing home's director of nursing offered to arrange meetings and keep everyone informed by e-mail. Three people agreed to look into a regional form for communicating decisions about CPR, and the group agreed to meet again at one of the nursing homes in a month.

This had the makings of real change. People were excited. They had bypassed the common diversions of spending too much time gathering information or putting all their efforts into standard "continuing education" work. Instead, they tried out two changes on a small scale. Based on what they learn, they will spread the useful changes more widely. They agreed on specific measures to monitor whether changes really improve things for patients. Within a month, they will have evidence of how their first two projects are working, they can make corrections in plans, and they can continue that work and start new projects.

Making Change Happen

The team working on the shared communication device quickly encountered stories of success from other regions, Oregon's Physician Orders for Life-Sustaining Treatment (POLST), for example (1). They adapted POLST and started the long process of getting agreement from legal authorities, community leaders, and health care organizations. That work got a major boost when the local newspaper ran a series on end-of-life care and highlighted the importance of this work. Remarkably, Dr. Thomas saw his first patient with a form adapted from the POLST just 4 months after Mrs. Harroldson's death.

The Coalition realized early that it needed to measure results. The rate of Do-Not-Resuscitate (DNR) orders in the minimum data set (standard data collection for nursing facilities) in five local nursing facilities went from 28% to 52% over 6 months, and the rate of those DNR orders being transferred to the hospital went from 2 in 12 transfers in the 3 months before the project to 6 in 8 transfers in a 3-month period starting 6 months later.

The team at the nursing home that offered to try out routine consideration of advance care planning had more problems. First, they found that patients had all sorts of pre-existing written advance directive documents which they and their families had not put in the nursing facility's records. Second, they found that their clinicians were not asking patients or families to make these decisions in advance. The care team realized that they really did not have much expertise or comfort with these discussions. A chaplain at a nearby hospital offered a training package on advance care planning and decision-making. They also asked a few family members to talk with them and learned that families would generally welcome the chance to talk about what their loved ones faced. By this point, an audit of the medical records at the facility showed that advance care plans of some sort were document-

ed for 12% of the patients at the initiation of the project and for 64% one year later. The team was delighted and surprised because it had run into so many problems that most felt that they were not really accomplishing much. All this took some months, but much was learned and most of it was shared widely through the Coalition's e-mail newsletter.

The variability of the process of change is obvious. Some issues move along quickly, and others require long struggles. The fact that both teams engineered some measures to monitor improvement turned out to be important. The teams will continue to collect data on these measures over time to test whether the changes are really improvements. Success requires keeping the pace of change visible, keeping the aim visible, and keeping powerful leaders supportive. The nursing home director could have shut down the process of improvement in advance planning at any time, just by voicing concern. Instead, she became an advocate because the aim was important and the team's approach was so effective. Most teams cannot sustain the effort needed to keep more than a few endeavors going at one time, but most can do that much. The most effective teams are "infectious," passing along to others the enthusiasm and the method by helping them get underway.

Reform in End-of-Life Care

During the past 30 years, end-of-life care has gradually improved, by at least some measures. The rate of use of opioids on a per capita basis has increased by more than tenfold (2). Cancer patients once were given neither their diagnosis nor effective pain relief. Now, virtually all get at least the diagnosis and basic pain treatment. Hospice has shown that better care is possible in targeted, dedicated, and comprehensive care systems. Fewer residents of nursing facilities have physical or chemical restraints, and advance directives are being more widely used to document patient choices.

Nevertheless, most efforts to improve care delivery have been ineffective. Much of the work in improving end-of-life care has focused on either 1) the pursuit of patient self-determination and engagement in decision-making, or 2) the pursuit of biomedical understanding and improved therapy.

The first endeavor has been highly visible but largely ineffective. The SUPPORT study tried to enable thousands of very sick patients to participate in decision-making and failed to change behaviors or outcomes (3). Most studies report that about one-fourth of seriously ill persons have a written advance directive before they die, and the most rigorous designs have not evidenced improvements in patient care on the basis of advance directives (4,5). The strongest determinant of locus of care at the time of death across regions is hospital bed availability and usage, not patient characteristics (6). The strongest determinant of DNR status is proximity to death (2).

Researchers and political leaders offer basic research as a mode of reform, and improved therapeutic options have contributed substantially to improved care. Still, most people who have serious pain do not need advanced methods; they just need the morphine and counseling that have been available for centuries. The failure of the care system to employ well-proven methods is stunning. Most patients with congestive heart failure do not receive the best drugs, and most do not know how to manage their illness (7). Most patients with asthma do not know how to use their inhalers (8,9). Research has created opportunities that are being squandered for lack of a focused system to implement better care.

Into this gap come common-sense efforts to improve care delivery, like Dr. Thomas's. Myriad providers are now setting out to hold themselves to stricter standards, to monitor performance, and to try out innovations.

In July 1997, the Institute for Healthcare Improvement (IHI) and the Center to Improve Care of the Dying (CICD) launched a year-long collaboration among teams from 48 provider organizations across the United States and Canada. With the guidance of experts and with sound methods for improvement, most found ways to make substantial improvements for their patients. One hospital-based team found, much to their chagrin, that the average cancer patient waited 3 hours for medication in response to pain. The reasons were many: routines, regulations, and other priorities. By working to improve and standardize assessment and treatment, the team within just a few months reduced the average response time to less than 1 hr (Fig. 13-1). Another team found that they could get medications to patients more quickly by authorizing an on-the-scene nurse to make adjustments within an agreed range. Many found that pain was simply being ignored, and they required measuring pain as "the fifth vital sign."

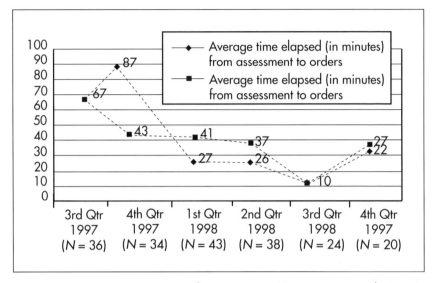

Figure 13-1. Response time to pain, by quarter-years. (Courtesy Jean Brontoli, SSM, St. Mary's Medical Center, St. Louis, MO).

One team virtually abolished severe and persistent dyspnea in a hospice population. Initially, half of the patients had troubling shortness of breath lasting more than 8 hr. They started prioritizing quick responses, having a physician-endorsed treatment protocol, a back-up physician if the attending physician did not respond or the problem persisted, and appropriate drugs in stock in the patient's home (ready to give with a phone call). The rate of troubling dyspnea lasting more than 8 hr fell to zero, within half a year (Fig. 13-2).

Many of the IHI-CICD collaborative teams worked to improve family support. Virtually every team that worked on family support made improvements that mattered. Some initiated bereavement support. Some tackled issues that made families angry or that demonstrated insensitivity in the system. Many hospitals, for example, were found to be sending the bill for the final hospital stay to the now-dead patient. Families found this to be one more piece of evidence that no one cared, but changing the computer address to "the estate of" was a help. Other teams worked on ensuring follow-up contact with family after a death. Two provided beepers to family caregivers at home or to families holding vigils in a hospital, so that they could be absent for a short sleep or to run errands without feeling out of touch. One provided a place for families to shower and nap while a loved one was in the hos-

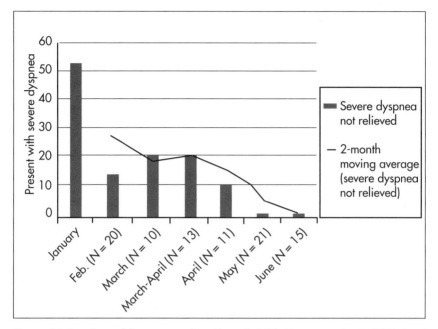

Figure 13-2. Rates of dyspnea not relieved by end of shift. (As presented at the IHI National Congress for End-of-Life Breakthrough Series, July 1998, Joan Teno, Lifespan, Rhode Island; courtesy Joan Teno.)

pital. Each of these projects identified specific measures to monitor the impact of the changes and were therefore able to show that the new approaches improved the experience for patients or families.

Franciscan Health System in Tacoma, Washington, initiated a clever and effective use of community volunteers. A skilled nurse (0.7 FTE), a chaplain (0.2 FTE), and a few concerned providers recruited local volunteers. Physicians identified patients in a general medicine clinic who were "sick enough to die in the next year." The team made sure these patients got the opportunity to make care plans for future care. Volunteers called these patients regularly, offered a friendly voice, and identified when things might be going badly. They then notified the nurse, who functioned as the care manager. Patients did better, used more community services, came into hospice earlier, had fewer hospitalizations, were more likely to die at home, and generated more hospice income, compared with patients identified in the same way at a similar clinic that did not have the special program (Figs. 13-3 to 13-5).

The collaborating teams improved their own programs and

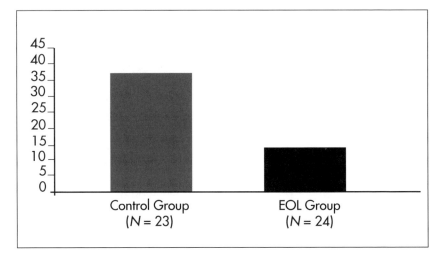

Figure 13-3. Number of hospitalizations in last year of life. (As presented at the IHI National Congress for the End-of-Life Breakthrough Series, July 1998, Franciscan Health System, Tacoma, WA; courtesy Franciscan Health System.)

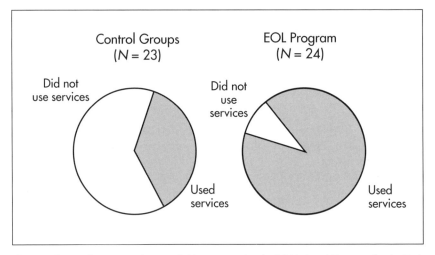

Figure 13-4. Support services used. (As presented at the IHI National Congress for the End-of-life Breakthrough Series, July 1998, by Franciscan Health System, Tacoma, WA; courtesy of Franciscan Health System.)

learned a number of generalizable insights (Table 13-1). For example, most practitioners use a "mental model" of having a long phase in the course of eventually fatal illness in which the dominant aim is to cure or substantially modify the time course of the illness. The mental model goes on to assume a short phase of "dying," in which the person clear-

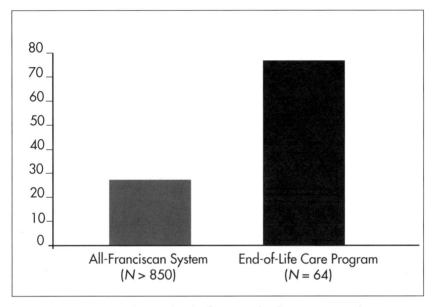

Figure 13-5. Average hospice length of stay. (Updated 6 August 1999 by Georganne Trandum, Franciscan Health System, Tacoma, WA; courtesy of Franciscan Health System.)

Table 13-1. Some Insights About Improving End-of-Life Care from the Breakthrough Series.

Identifying the population
   Not "Who is dying?" but "Who is sick enough that it would not be suprising if he or she died within a few months or a year?"
Advance planning
   Most potential emergencies can be anticipated, planned, rehearsed, and rendered "routine," including physical aspects of care near death.
Pain and other symptoms
   Prevent symptoms and fear with routine assessment, aggressive preventive treatment, and prompt response.
Transfers
   Prevent commonplace calamities by having medications, Do-Not-Resuscitate orders, advance care plans, and family education continue across transfers.
Meaningfulness
   Ask "If you were to die soon, what would be left undone?" Then help the patient do those things.

ly loses ground and during which treatments should be aimed at comfort. The "trick" is to identify the "just right" time at which to "switch from cure to care" (10). Of course, this is notoriously difficult. Recent evidence shows, for example, that the average person who dies of congestive heart failure today had at least a 50-50 chance to live 6 months just yesterday (11). Even with colon and lung cancer, the median chance to survive 2 months is more than 20% on the day before death and almost 50% 1 week earlier.

Thus, many patients will die shortly after having had an ambiguous prognosis (12). When our teams first tried to identify "dying" patients at whom to target their interventions, few patients were named by physicians, and then only very late in their course. It seemed that physicians had learned to identify people late enough that the prognosis was never seriously wrong. Teams learned instead to identify patients to target for special services with what we now call the "surprise" question. We asked physicians to identify those who "were sick enough that it would not be surprising if he or she died in the next 6 months." Interestingly, it did not matter much whether we asked about a few months or a year. The point is that the question now encourages physicians to note that the patient is very sick and makes clear that it is expected that some who are "sick enough to die" will still live a long time. Using this approach, many more patients were identified far enough ahead of death to make a difference in their lives by having access to hospice and other end-of-life services. We are learning that many patients identified this way choose to receive aggressive life-sustaining treatment, not "palliative care *only*." This underscores the importance of avoiding the false dichotomy of a transition from "cure to care."

The collaborative quality improvement endeavor reported here illustrates a promising trend toward multisite, coordinated improvement projects. The Decisions Near the End-of-Life project (*http://www.edc.org/CAE/Decisions/dnel.html*), coordinated by EDC in Newton, Massachusetts, in conjunction with the American Hospital Association and the Hastings Center, has provided support and interaction between dozens of hospitals. The Maine Hospital Association is coordinating support for 24 hospitals working to improve the end of life. The Veteran's Administration joined IHI and CICD in another collaboration among 36 teams addressing advanced heart and lung failure (13).

Regional excellence might result from intense local collaboration. A few years ago, before the collaborative process reported above, the major health care providers of La Crosse, Wisconsin, embarked upon a community-wide effort to improve advance care planning (14). In a remarkable collaboration, they instructed elderly persons in senior centers, patients when coming to office visits, and ordinary citizens receiving the news through the mass media. They expanded their vision from legal forms for advance directives to comprehensive advance care planning, aiming to anticipate possible emergencies and to articulate preferences about how the end of life would be lived. In the only such population-based analysis to date, 85% of more than 500 decedents had an advance directive at the time of death, and that directive that had been written, on average, more than a year ahead of death. In La Crosse, 98% of dying people had deliberately forgone some treatment, and virtually all of the advance directives were followed. How did the providers accomplish this? They had a few teams with common goals and they supported them through an array of interventions, assessments, and broader implementation of the efforts that worked.

Rapid Quality Improvement

The barrier facing improvement teams is often getting any change started. Associates in Process Improvement and others have designed an effective and useful method of rapidly initiating changes (15,16). The Model for Improvement starts with teams asking themselves three fundamental questions:

1. What are we trying to accomplish? (Aim)
2. How will we know that a change is an improvement? (Measure)
3. What changes can we make? (Changes)

These questions can be addressed in any order, so long as the answers are coherent.

What are we trying to accomplish? The answer to this question formulates the goal of the team and helps to guide and focus the overall improvement effort. Compelling aims are usually brief, measurable, and important to patients and families. The aim should be documented and circulated for comment to those who have a stake in the work or the outcome of the project.

How will we know that a change is an improvement? Measurement is an important part of the improvement process, allowing teams to quantify the impact of changes and determine whether or not the changes actually lead to improvement. Measurement should provide answers to specific questions. For example, did instituting a protocol reduce the incidence of pain? Did the provision of written information, reminders, and the tools to manage exacerbations at home prevent families from making unnecessary emergency room visits? Measurement should be used to determine whether specific aims are being achieved.

What changes can we make? People directly involved with a malfunctioning process often have suggestions. Patients, families, providers, and managers will have thoughts on "what would work better." Review of the literature and of the experiences of others often reveals changes that are well-tested but not extensively used in practice.

With these questions answered, teams move quickly to testing the most appealing changes using the Plan-Do-Study-Act (PDSA) cycle.

The Plan-Do-Study-Act Cycle

The model for improvement is based on a trial and learning approach. The PDSA cycle provides the framework for effectuating change by planning it, trying it, observing the consequences, then acting on what is learned from those consequences. All four steps are important. All too often, a change is tried but not evaluated, and nothing useful is learned.

The changes identified from a successful project often must be adapted to the local setting. This may require a few PDSA cycles. Even an ambitious and innovative change can be tested first on a small scale, for example, with only one or two physicians, with the next five patients, for the next three days, or one component at a time. Small scale refers only to the scope of a particular cycle. The change that is eventually implemented could well be a significant departure from current practice. This approach overcomes some of the reasons for inactivity: the risks involved, resources, and the lack of confidence that the change will work.

Measurement of effect is critical to learning in tests. The most convincing measures are those documented in a time series, for example, the percentage of clinic patients each month who have had an advanced care planning discussion, or the average response time for pain relief on the oncology unit each week. The temporal relationship between changes made and the results builds evidence that the changes led to improvement. Even the size of the sample can vary because changes are refined and data is collected over time. The team should aim to have just enough evidence to assess whether changes result in improvements and to sustain the changes that work.

Sometimes it is enough to measure "before" and "after" or "intervention" and "control." If such a measurement strategy is used, additional qualitative assessments regarding the impact of the changes help innovators learn from each cycle and refine the changes.

Testing multiple changes with dozens of teams during the collaborative quality improvement provides an opportunity to learn complex system behavior quickly. Those insights can build a platform for other organizations interested in improving care at the end of life (17).

Quality Improvement in Relation to Conventional Research

In science today, carefully designed randomized experiments and tests of hypotheses are often the only trusted avenues to gaining knowledge. Other formal research methods, such as case-control and cohort studies, can also provide reliable insights. However, the art of medical care involves a continuing, individualized search in which the physician tries to match incomplete scientific knowledge of disease and treatment with incomplete knowledge about particular patients and local care systems. Physicians do not often know the way but find it step by step, inductively learning from experience reflected upon and informed by their care of real patients. Often, steady investigation with small-scale tests of change are more useful than the traditional, randomized, controlled clinical trial in discerning how to care for a particular population. The alternative to using a sequence of PDSA cycles and data plotted over time is not usually a randomized trial followed by widespread implementation; it is usually continuing present practices or making changes without evidence or evaluation.

PDSA cycles linked to important aims and thoughtful reflection are powerful tools for learning in complex systems when the goal is to improve those systems. Practice patterns vary widely in every medical discipline across the country (18). For example, rates of breast-conserving surgery for breast cancer vary more than 30-fold in the United States (19). Similarly, most elderly persons with myocardial infarction do not receive beta-blocker therapy in their post-acute management (20). Rates of cesarean section range from 8% to more than 40% among hospital service areas (21). Variations in practice patterns are so great that not all practitioners can be right, and PDSA approaches can guide reform. The PDSA method can catalyze change in a system that is performing poorly relative to its potential.

When we are uncertain about the benefit of a particular drug or operation relative to that of its alternatives, no investigatory design can yield a more confident conclusion than the randomized, controlled trial. But the same is not true when we are trying to develop an improved patient flow or when we are trying to adapt a specific treatment or flowchart for use in a local setting.

Indeed, most learning and improvement in real-world settings comes neither from erratic trial and error nor from randomized experiments but from PDSA science (15). The work of the Northern New England Cardiovascular Disease Study Group in the late 1980s and early 1990s (22) studied variations in outcomes and processes of care among participating centers. Physicians played a leadership role in trying to make this variation informative. Round-robin visiting among surgical teams, with linkage to a voluntary database on surgical outcomes and complications, allowed clinical groups to identify promising changes in numerous components of cardiovascular surgery, including patient selection, preoperative preparation, bypass pump management, hemostasis, and anesthesia. This rich array of observations, often arising in regular meetings of the group, led to numerous local PDSA cycles, the results of which were reported back to the group as a whole. The overall result, achieved without a randomized trial but with many disciplined cycles of reflection and action, was a 24% decline in mortality from coronary artery bypass graft surgery throughout the region. This dramatic change probably could not have been achieved using a formal, large-scale, randomized trial.

Lessons to Learn

Dr. Thomas and the group members did many things right:

- Dr. Thomas took responsibility and got things started.
- He got the right people involved, including senior leaders.

- The group members took on situations that they could improve and that affected patients.
- They used existing knowledge as the basis for developing their changes.
- They adapted existing tools and skills from other areas to their own needs.
- They measured results over time.
- They started small (just one nursing facility) for the tougher problems and built knowledge about the changes sequentially.
- Their successes catalyzed larger changes and an attitude of welcoming innovation and improvement.

Summary

The time is right for innovation and changes in end-of-life care, all guided by measurement and catalyzed by effective networking among innovators. Rapid cycle quality improvement offers leverage for change that reformers can respect and utilize. We need multifaceted change that aims for consistent high-value and high-quality care and better understanding of the nature of good end-of-life care. To meet this challenge and be prepared for the groundswell of need in our aging population, we must harness our resources and commit to these efforts now. Each of us must ask *What shortcomings in end-of-life care exist? How can they be addressed? How will improvement be accomplished?* And, most importantly, *What can I improve, this week, in my health care system?*

REFERENCES

1 The Physician Orders for Life-Sustaining Treatment (POLST). Available from OHSU Center for Ethics in Health Care via the Internet (http://www.ohsu.edu/ethics/polst.htm). Accessed on 6 Aug. 1999.
2 **Robert Wood Johnson Foundation.** State Initiatives in End-of-life Care: Using Qualitative and Quantitative Data to Shape Policy Change. Issue 1. June 1998.
3. **The SUPPORT Principal Investigators.** A controlled trial to improve care for seriously ill hospitalized patients: The Study to Understand Prognoses and Preferences for Outcomes and Risks of Treatments (SUPPORT). JAMA. 1995;274:1591-8.

4. **Teno JM, Licks S, Lynn J, et al for the SUPPORT Investigators.** Do advance directives provide instructions that direct care? J Am Geriatr Soc. 1997;45:508-12.

5. **Schneiderman LJ, Pearlman RA, Kaplan RM, et al.** Relationship of general advance directive instructions to specific life-sustaining treatment preferences in patients with serious illness. Arch Intern Med. 1992;152:2114-22.

6. **Pritchard RS, Fisher ES, Teno JM, et al for the SUPPORT investigators.** Influence of patient preferences and local health system characteristics on the place of death. J Am Geriatr Soc. 1998;46:1242-50.

7. **Rich MW.** Heart failure disease management: a critical review. J Card Fail. 1999;1:64-75.

8. **Bailey WC, Richards JM, Brooks CM, et al.** A randomized trial to improve self-management practices of adults with asthma. Arch Intern Med. 1990;150:1664-8.

9. **Epstein SW, Manning CD, Ashley MJ, Corey PN.** Survey of the clinical use of hand-held inhalers. Cancer Med Assoc J. 1979;120:813-6.

10. **Callahan D.** Troubled Dream of Life. New York: Simon & Schuster; 1993.

11. **Lynn J, Harrell F, Cohn F, et al.** Prognoses of seriously ill hospitalized patients on the days before death: implications for patient care and public policy. New Horiz. 1997; 5:56-61.

12. **Lynn J.** An 88-year-old woman facing the end of life. JAMA. 1997;277:1633-40.

13. **Lynn J, Schall M, Milne C, et al.** Quality improvements in end of life care: insights from two quality improvement collaboratives. Jt Comm J Qual Improv. 2000;26:254-67.

14. **Hammes BJ, Rooney BL.** Death and end-of-life planning in one midwestern community. Arch Intern Med. 1998;158:383-90.

15. **Berwick DM.** Developing and testing changes in delivery of care. Ann Intern Med. 1998;128:651-6.

16. **Langley G, Nolan K, Nolan T, et al.** The Improvement Book. San Francisco: Jossey-Bass; 1996.

17. **Lynn J, Schuster JL.** Improving Care at the End of Life: A Sourcebook for Health Care Managers and Clinicians. New York: Oxford University Press; forthcoming.

18. The Dartmouth Atlas of Health Care. Chicago: American Hospital Publishing; 1996.

19. **Lazovich, DA, White, E, Thomas, DB, Moe, RE.** Underutilization of breast-conserving surgery and radiation therapy among women with stage I or II breast cancer. JAMA. 1991;266:3433-8.

20. **Soumerai SB, McLauglin TJ, Spiegelman D, et al.** Adverse outcomes of underuse of beta-blockers in elderly survivors of acute myocardial infarction. JAMA. 1997;277:115-21.

21. **Sandmire HF, DeMott RK.** The Green Bay cesarean section study III: falling cesarean birth rates without a formal curtailment program. Am J Obstet Gynecol. 1994;170:1790-9.

22. **O'Connor GT, Plume SK, Olmstead EM, et al.** A regional intervention to improve the hospital mortality associated with coronary artery bypass graft surgery. The Northern New England Cardiovascular Disease Study Group. JAMA. 1996;275:841-6.

INDEX

Treatment, withdrawal of, 139-140
  legal issues of, 200
Tricyclic antidepressants
  for complicated grief, 189
  for depression in terminally ill,
    111, 113*t*, 114
Trust
  among African-American commu-
    nity, 49-52
  culturally effective care strategies
    for, 43*t*

U

Urgent care response, 227

V

Values
  cultural differences in with elderly
    Korean patient, 47-49

culturally effective care strategies
  for conflicts of, 43*t*
in decision-making process, 32-33
eliciting patient concerns about, 5-
  6
Vasopressors, forgoing, 148
Ventilatory support
  recommendations to discontinue,
    147
  withdrawal of, 148, 150-152, 154-
    155
Veterans Affairs, Department of, 228
Visiting policies, suspending of
  restrictions on, 154
Volume depletion, 130

W

Whole-brain radiation, 59
World Health Organization analgesic
  ladder, 77, 79